Eat to Beat Low Blood Sugar

Eat to Beat Low Blood Sugar

The Nutritional Plan to Overcome Hypoglycaemia, with 60 recipes

Martin Budd *and*
Maggie Budd

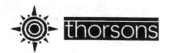

Thorsons
An Imprint of HarperCollins*Publishers*
77–85 Fulham Palace Road
Hammersmith, London W6 8JB

The website address is:
www.thorsonselement.com

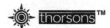

and *Thorsons*
are trademarks of
HarperCollins*Publishers* Limited

Published by Thorsons 2003

A catalogue record for this book
is available from the British Library

ISBN **978 0 00 714788 5**

Find out more about HarperCollins and the environment at
www.harpercollins.co.uk/green

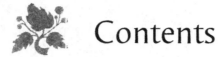

Contents

Introduction

Since the publication of my first book, *Low Blood Sugar*, in 1981, the established medical attitude to the diagnosis and treatment of low blood sugar has radically changed. For many years doctors viewed sudden falls in the blood sugar as a relatively harmless cause of the sort of transient symptoms that we can all at times experience. The recommended treatment at the time was usually sugar cubes or a bar of chocolate.

These days, low blood sugar, or hypoglycaemia to give it its proper name, is seen by many doctors, naturopaths and researchers as an important clue that indicates a general inefficiency in our sugar regulation system. This faulty control has been termed dysglycaemia.

A host of symptoms and health problems are now known to develop as a result of poor blood sugar regulation. These include obesity, high blood pressure, anxiety, depression, fatigue, late onset diabetes, gout, heart disease, thyroid and adrenal deficiency and a recently defined group of abnormalities known as Syndrome X, or the metabolic syndrome.

While some of the technical aspects of the diagnosis and treatment of low blood sugar will be briefly discussed, this book essentially offers dietary advice to readers with low blood sugar to enable them to help themselves. Correct eating to minimize the adverse effects of dysglycaemia can reduce the distressing symptoms of low blood sugar, and lessen the risk of the many health problems associated with a high sugar diet that can develop in later life.

Part One looks at what low blood sugar means, its causes and symptoms. Part Two concerns itself with diet, providing guidance on what you should and should not be eating and the importance of timing meals well, as well as an easy-to-follow low blood sugar diet. Low blood sugar can cause a wide range of problems and the solution is not always the same. For this reason, a range of case histories is provided to illustrate some of the problems and solutions involved.

Part Three is where we get practical with the *Eat to Beat Low Blood Sugar* recipes. Here you will find a selection of recipes appropriate for a low blood sugar diet – both in terms of their content and when they are designed to be eaten. Part Four, entitled Taking it Further, outlines the value of specific nutritional supplements used to treat low blood sugar.

Towards the end of the book you will also find a glossary that explains the terminology currently in use in the field of blood sugar imbalances – for instance, Syndrome X, insulin resistance, glycaemic index and dysglycaemia. Please note, low blood sugar, low blood glucose and hypoglycaemia are one and the same, so in order to avoid confusion I describe the condition as low blood sugar throughout this book.

PART ONE

Low Blood Sugar – Facts and Figures

CHAPTER 1

So what exactly is low blood sugar?

Low blood 'sugar' refers to a low level of glucose in the blood. There are no rigid criteria for diagnosing low blood sugar, as considerable individual variations can exist. However, a blood glucose level of below 3.5mmol/litre will usually cause the typical symptoms of low blood sugar. This is not a rare condition – everyone reading this book will have experienced the symptoms of low blood sugar at some time in their lives.

However, for such a widespread problem, it is surprisingly misunderstood. Indeed for many people almost every aspect of the low blood sugar condition is either contradictory or confusing. This is well demonstrated by the questions that I am frequently asked, examples being:

- ✳ 'If diabetics with high blood sugar need to avoid sugar, why do those with low blood sugar also need to avoid sugar?'
- ✳ 'Why are the symptoms and causes of low blood sugar on the increase, yet most of us eat too much sugar?'
- ✳ 'Why do many people with low blood sugar develop high blood sugar [type II diabetes] in later life?'
- ✳ 'My doctor has advised me to suck a sugar cube whenever I feel shaky or dizzy between meals [low blood sugar symptoms]. You advise me to avoid sugar, who is correct and why?'
- ✳ 'We are told that all the carbohydrates in our diet end up as glucose in the blood. Do I therefore need to avoid all forms of carbohydrate for the remainder of my life?'

The answers to these and other questions will become apparent as you read this book.

The beginning – the discovery of low blood sugar
Perhaps low blood sugar should be termed 'Seale Harris Syndrome' after the American GP who first defined its symptoms in 1924. Dr Harris – a contemporary of Banting and Best, the co-discoverers of the role of insulin in diabetes – noticed that many diabetic patients attending the new insulin clinics developed symptoms of *low* blood sugar.

Given that diabetes is characterized by a *high* blood sugar level, caused by the lack of insulin (a hormone that controls the level of glucose in the blood), this observation was surprising. The reason, however, was simple – many diabetics have difficulty in accurately judging their insulin requirements and often overdose themselves, producing a condition known as hyperinsulinism, which consequently causes low blood sugar (or hypo).

Crucially, Dr Harris noted that he also had several patients in his regular practice who exhibited symptoms of the 'hypo' reaction on a regular basis, but who were *not* diabetic and were therefore not taking insulin. He accurately concluded that these patients probably experienced the unpleasant symptoms of hypoglycaemia as a result of an inefficiency or imbalance in their sugar-regulating apparatus. This complex mechanism involves the islet glands of the pancreas that release insulin, the liver, to some extent the pituitary, thyroid and adrenal glands and other functions that play a part in sugar metabolism.

Dr Harris discussed his ideas with Dr Banting, who agreed that the role of insulin in non-diabetic low blood sugar offered a new aspect to the study of blood sugar balance. No papers on the topic had appeared in medical literature prior to Seale Harris's work, but his discoveries led to numerous similar papers appearing in journals all over the world.

CHAPTER 2

The causes of low blood sugar

You may ask why many people who eat and drink excessive amounts of sugar-rich foods do not suffer from low blood sugar, while others who follow a near-perfect low sugar diet experience low blood sugar symptoms. The answer appears to lie in the many background health influences that can predispose an individual to dysglycaemia and low blood sugar.

This is a very complex subject but a brief list will serve to highlight the chief causative factors:

* Excessive sugar intake, leading to pancreatic overstimulation, hyperinsulinism and insulin resistance.
* Adrenal under-production, leading to adrenal deficiency or hypoadrenalism.
* Imbalance and subsequent deficiency of the thyroid.
* Excessive use of tobacco (each cigarette smoked raises the blood sugar equivalent to $2\frac{1}{2}$ teaspoons of sugar).
* Excessive use of alcohol and caffeine – both serve to stress the adrenal mechanism.
* Inability to handle prolonged or excessive stress, leading to adrenal debility and inefficiency (known in the US as adrenal exhaustion or adrenal fatigue).
* Food allergies or intolerances, which can be caused by, but also aggravated by, low blood sugar.
* Mineral deficiencies. These include chromium, which is now deficient in the soil of Western nations. The minerals zinc, vanadium, magnesium, manganese and potassium are also essential for optimum blood sugar control.
* Hereditary factors, in particular a family history of diabetes, hypothyroidism, asthma, epilepsy, clinical depression or chronic fatigue.

When attempting to treat blood sugar disorders one key question that must always be considered is whether the patient's low blood sugar is only a symptom, or is itself a cause of symptoms.

Fasting hypoglycaemia

When low blood sugar is simply a symptom, it is generally the result of fasting, or transient, hypoglycaemia – low blood sugar that is caused by a delayed or missed meal. This is something we have all experienced; the symptoms include shakiness or dizziness and fatigue, perhaps a mild headache or a feeling of ill temper. Usually the symptoms are coupled with a strong urge for chocolate or something sweet.

Those who experience such symptoms on waking each morning usually have a background health problem. However, there are very few health problems that can cause us to feel worse on rising than we feel upon retiring. The list includes adrenal exhaustion, hypothyroidism, drug addiction and alcoholism. Those with severe food intolerances can also feel tired, thickheaded and irritable on waking – the reason for this is thought to be the early onset of withdrawal symptoms resulting from the night fast.

Reactive, or functional, hypoglycaemia

This problem is the main subject of this book. It defines a type of chronic low blood sugar that usually requires an appropriate dietary strategy and supplement use. The symptoms can occur at any time and, for many unfortunate sufferers, can be virtually continuous.

WHAT HAPPENS TO THE BLOOD?

The symptoms of low blood sugar can develop as a result of two principle changes in the blood sugar. These changes can involve either the actual low level of the blood sugar or the speed of fall in the blood sugar. Unfortunately the human brain cannot store glucose, so even a five per cent fall in the available glucose supply to the brain and nervous system can produce an adrenal response with subsequent symptoms.

WHAT ARE THE IDEAL GLUCOSE LEVELS?

The normal level of our fasting blood sugar (fasting refers to food avoidance for 12 hours) is 4–7mmol/L. Many diabetic clinics define a patient's symptoms as 'hypo' if a patient's blood falls below 4mmol/L. However, I have frequently seen great symptom variations in a patient's response to low blood sugar levels, although generally I have found that a blood sugar level below 3.5mmol/L can predictably cause symptoms to surface.

The American doctor and nutritionist Carlton Fredericks, a renowned authority on low blood sugar, stated 'when blood sugar drops as little as 0.25mmol/L below *the normal for the patient*, a profound glandular compensation may start'. However, as mentioned above, a low level of blood sugar is not the only cause of low blood sugar symptoms – an inappropriately rapid *fall* in the blood glucose can also give rise to symptoms.

SPEED OF FALL IN BLOOD SUGAR

A rapid fall in the blood sugar level (for whatever reason) in excess of 1.5mmol/L in one hour can produce symptoms of low blood sugar. These changes occur irrespective of the actual level of blood sugar, for example a fall from 7mmol/L to 5mmol/L in 30–45 minutes can often cause low blood sugar symptoms to develop.

Both of the trigger factors that cause low blood sugar symptoms – i.e. speed of fall and a general low level – are subject to individual variations. I have seen patients who appeared to be symptom-free with a blood sugar level of 2.5mmol/L and others with levels around 3.5mmol/L who could barely walk or talk.

Insulin-dependent diabetics can 'hypo' when they overdose on their insulin requirements in relation to food and/or activity. Glucometers are used to check their blood glucose levels. Early models were designed to measure high blood sugar levels, however the more recent glucometers can measure blood sugar levels as low as 1.5mmol/L with a finger-prick blood sample. Accurate results can be achieved within 6–60 seconds, depending on the model used.

The problems caused by too much sugar

The high-carbohydrate Western diet provides sugar far in excess of our energy needs. Consumption of sugar alone in Great Britain amounts to 27kg (60–65lb) per person per year. If you include the sugar-rich refined carbohydrates we eat (for example, sweets, chocolates, cookies, cakes, cereals, soda and cola drinks) then our total sugar 'load' can be as high as 90kg (200lbs) per person (the figures in the US follow close behind). In terms of calories, one teaspoon of sugar per day equals 100 calories per week, so the amount of calories consumed by someone at the top end of the sugar-intake scale is vast.

When we eat sugar, we either use it for energy needs, or it is stored as glycogen or fat. Marathon runners know that they need to consume extra carbohydrates three to four days before a race to provide stored fuel for gradual release during the race. Likewise, those who do heavy manual work can often avoid weight and health problems as a result of converting all their food (fuel) directly to energy.

The experience of the explorer Sir Ranulph Fiennes clearly demonstrates how important it is that we match our energy intake to our output. On an Arctic trek, Fiennes lost weight despite consuming 5000 calories a day. In spite of his high calorie diet, his energy requirements meant he utilized a total of 11,000 calories each day. His subsequent weight loss was therefore inevitable. Perhaps we could justify our high sugar diets with marathon running or polar exploration – not popular choices. Fortunately there are other solutions (these are discussed in Part Two).

Insulin

Central to the problem of low blood sugar is the hormone insulin. Any rise in our blood sugar requires an insulin response. Insulin is a hormone secreted by the pancreas to lower blood glucose levels; it does this by transporting the glucose to the muscle cells and other tissues. Insulin is uniquely the only hormone to promote food (fuel) storage for future use. For this reason it is often termed the storage or fattening hormone.

This storage facility was essential for human survival several thousand years ago, for the early hunter-gatherers were very similar to the present day big cat carnivores in Africa and India. Their eating habits consisted of large meals perhaps every three to four days. The ability to store food was therefore a vital survival strategy. Unfortunately 21st-century men and women follow a largely sedentary lifestyle yet they often eat carbohydrate-rich meals and snacks three to six times daily. Our metabolism can only convert a small amount of excessive sugar to glycogen, which is stored in the liver and muscle cells. The remainder is stored as fat. Our food is our fuel and if the fuel is not required it is stored and excess weight is the result.

However, a sugar-laden diet does not only lead to the storage of fat. Because the insulin response is constantly being overworked, it can become less efficient as the cells become less sensitive and resistant to the effect of the insulin.

INSULIN RESISTANCE

This gradual loss of sensitivity to the blood insulin results in an increase in the level of insulin as the pancreas secretes more and more in an attempt to normalize the blood sugar balance. The end result is an on-going high level of blood insulin (hyper-insulinaemia). This excess insulin promotes more fat storage at the expense of available energy. High-sugar and high-carbohydrate eating can eventually lead to obesity, high blood fats, high blood pressure and fatigue (this group of disorders is known as Syndrome X, or metabolic syndrome). Such inappropriately high levels of blood insulin can cause chronic irritable bowel syndrome, adrenal exhaustion and disturbances to the female hormonal balance (as in Polycystic Ovary Syndrome).

The adrenal response

Although the brain and nervous system rely on blood sugar as the chief nutrient, excessively high levels of blood sugar can cause damage to nerve cells.

The temporary fall in the blood sugar caused by the insulin response to food triggers adrenal compensation, where adrenaline is released to counter the effect of the low blood sugar. This yo-yoing of the blood sugar levels can lead to a chronic imbalance in the blood sugar control (dysglycaemia), causing adrenal deficiency and a reduced thyroid hormone output. The thyroid gland reflects our metabolic rate and mild hypothyroidism can result from adrenal exhaustion.

The role of the adrenal hormone adrenaline in the blood sugar narrative highlights a design fault in our body chemistry. This vital hormone has two major functions. These are stress-handling (the so-called fight or flight response) and raising our blood sugar when the level falls too low.

As any athlete knows, adrenaline increases the metabolic rate, the heart rate, the blood flow to muscles and the oxygen intake. In a primitive society this would prepare us to either run or attack. However, for those of us who suffer from low blood sugar (which causes our brain and nervous system efficiency to be compromised), the adrenaline response that occurs is identical to our reaction to any type of stress. This explains why so many sufferers of long-term low blood sugar experience episodes of aggression and mood changes – examples being women with pre-menstrual syndrome and diabetics or non-diabetics who 'hypo'. Our metabolism cannot identify the *reason* for the adrenal surge, hence the stress response that occurs with low blood sugar.

Summary

The modern high carbohydrate/sugar diet, coupled with our sedentary lifestyle, has lead to an increase in many low blood sugar symptoms, including obesity, fatigue and poor stress handling. The subsequent adrenal compensation and exhaustion can result in mild hypothyroidism, high blood pressure and subsequently Syndrome X. Anxiety, depression, elevated blood fats and metabolic depression can be the consequence.

In the next chapter we look at the many symptoms that can result from low blood sugar.

CHAPTER 3

The symptoms of low blood sugar

One of the main problems in accurately diagnosing low blood sugar is that many of the symptoms of the condition can have other causes.

General symptoms and problems

To discuss the diversity of symptoms caused by low blood sugar would take up most of this book. However, the list below is a representative selection of the most common symptoms that can be caused in part or wholly by low blood sugar.

Fatigue	Anxiety	Depression
Irritability	Forgetfulness	Poor concentration
Indigestion	Breathlessness	Panic feelings
Headaches	Migraine	Asthma
Overweight	Food cravings	Excessive smoking
Alcoholism	Vertigo	Sweating
Pre-menstrual tension	Muscular stiffness	Phobias
Numbness	Blurred vision	Cold extremities
Joint pain	Fainting and blackouts	Convulsions
Nightmares	Lack of sex drive	Allergies
Angina	Suicidal tendencies	Irritable bowel symptoms
Epilepsy	Stomach cramps	Stomach ulcers
Hyperactivity	Neuralgia	Agoraphobia
Narcolepsy	Tinnitus	

I am sure there will be many eyebrows raised at the great variety and number of symptoms I have listed and, at first sight, it is difficult to imagine that there is a common theme to all these conditions.

Interestingly though, many of the symptoms of low blood sugar are classed by doctors as 'stress disorders' and I hope to show, by describing the effect of sugar on the nervous system, that many of these symptoms are in fact due to nutritional imbalances and not 'personality failings'. You may see several of your own symptoms on the list; but simply to scan this list, recognize your symptoms and blame low blood sugar is not the answer. As previously stated, many of these symptoms may have other causes, not least of which could be stress.

Self-diagnosis is therefore not advisable; a naturopath or sympathetic doctor should be able to offer more objective diagnostic methods. These can include, in addition to detailed case-history taking, the six-hour glucose tolerance test, the measurement of adrenal and thyroid hormones and a blood insulin test (these will be discussed in due course).

At some time in their lives most people experience one or more of the symptoms listed above. They are usually caused by transient low blood sugar – a temporary or passing fall in the blood sugar level. This is rapidly rectified by the body's own sugar regulation mechanism. Once a balance is achieved, the symptoms usually disappear. If, however, there is a chronic imbalance in our sugar regulation, the symptoms may well improve or change, but they will always return if the actual imbalance is not corrected.

Now let us look more closely at the way in which a drop in the blood sugar directly affects the various organs and systems of the body, giving rise to the symptoms outlined. In this way you will begin to understand why the blood sugar level is so important to the normal running of the body. The effects of low blood sugar can be classified as follows:

Nervous system changes

The main nutrient needed by the nervous system is glucose. There is no really adequate substitute and, although other substances are involved, they cannot replace glucose. Unfortunately, it is not fully understood just how glucose acts on the nervous system, but it has been noted that when a healthy patient is injected with insulin (the opposite of glucose), profound and sudden changes in the efficiency of the nervous system occur within minutes. This is completely reversed by an injection of glucose. This tends to confirm that the nervous system requires a continuous supply of glucose in order to function efficiently.

Although the weight of an adult brain is only two per cent of the total body weight, the activity of the brain, in terms of utilization of glucose, may amount to 20–25 per cent of the total body activity. In spite of this, the total amount of glucose concentrated within the brain at any one time would, under normal conditions, be exhausted in 10–15 minutes. The effects of glucose starvation on the brain and nerve tissue as a result of a low level of blood sugar are as follows:

1 Insufficient oxygen.
2 Reduction in specific substances within the brain that are essential for nervous activity.

Let us look at the symptoms that can result from such changes.

CIRCULATORY CHANGES

Not surprisingly, the system first affected by a drop in the blood sugar level is the blood circulatory system. This, of course, includes the heart and blood vessels. When the blood sugar falls, the body automatically reacts in an attempt to restore balance to the system. This response involves the release of adrenaline from the adrenal glands, to raise the blood sugar. Adrenaline is also released in stressful situations. This means that if an individual has persistent low blood sugar, they may have symptoms similar to those produced by chronic stress. These can include:

1 An irregular increase in the heart rate, causing palpitations and breathing difficulties.
2 Angina-like symptoms involving a reduction in circulation to the heart muscle, chest cramp and pain in the chest and arms.
3 A general withdrawal of blood to deal with the 'stress effects', causing coldness of the hands and feet, muscular cramp and a poor adaptation to temperature changes.

GLANDULAR CHANGES

The changes involved in the glandular system following a drop in the blood sugar level are widespread and could well provide sufficient material for another book. However, in this context, it is adequate simply to briefly look at the glands affected.

1 Pituitary gland. This is the master control gland influencing the thyroid and adrenal glands.
2 Adrenal glands. These glands produce adrenaline, cortisol (hydrocortisone), DHEA and other hormones. It is the persistent stimulation of these glands in a patient suffering from low blood sugar that provides the causative link between blood sugar and rheumatoid arthritis. Overactivity, with subsequent exhaustion of the adrenal glands, can cause a reduction in the availability of cortisol and the 'mother' hormone DHEA, which provide protection against joint pain and inflammation.
3 Thyroid gland. Changes that occur with thyroid activity are of less significance than other glands. Although, like the adrenal and pituitary glands, the thyroid secretions are essentially antagonistic to insulin and thus thyroid imbalance can contribute to a blood sugar imbalance. A vicious cycle may be established whereby a mildly deficient thyroid causes low blood sugar and the subsequent adrenal stress can further depress the thyroid.

DIGESTIVE CHANGES

The changes in gastric (stomach) activity that occur with low blood sugar are mainly caused by the increased insulin level in the blood, rather than the actual deficiency of blood sugar. A standard hospital test to assess the efficiency of digestive activity involves administering to the patient an injection of insulin. This prompts a rapid and predictable increase in the amount of stomach acids, which are then measured. It follows that if this test has such an effect, the fluctuations of the insulin level in the blood – as occurs in low blood sugar and insulin resistance – would have a similar effect. Indeed, in practice, I find that many patients suffering from stomach ulcers, heartburn, hiatus hernia and other digestive ailments frequently have an underlying blood sugar imbalance.

Those with food intolerances may suffer symptoms that are partially caused by low blood sugar. Unfortunately, as a result of symptom similarity the two conditions are often confused.

PSYCHOLOGICAL CHANGES

As I discussed previously, changes in blood sugar can have a significant impact on the brain and nervous system – it is hardly surprising then that many patients suffering from low blood sugar also have personality problems. The most common symptoms found in low blood sugar patients are depression, anxiety and mental confusion. Many researchers, particularly in the US, consider chronic low blood sugar to be a contributing factor in such serious personality problems as schizophrenia and manic depression (bipolar disorder).

We know that low blood sugar can lead to fatigue of the adrenal glands, and that the adrenal glands are the body's main defence mechanism against stress. It therefore seems likely that those with chronic low blood sugar can suffer a vicious circle of adrenal exhaustion, which causes anxiety, and with the anxiety comes further exhaustion and stress. Unfortunately, many people suffering from stress often overeat or comfort-eat the wrong foods. They also tend to miss meals, relying on caffeine, tobacco and alcohol for their fuel, thus further aggravating any blood sugar imbalance.

Respiratory changes

Surprising as it may seem, low blood sugar can also affect the respiratory system. The reason for this is a substance called histamine. This compound is naturally present in all the cells of the body and has a variety of uses – not least is its role in controlling osmosis (passage of water) between the body membranes. It is well known that if the histamine level increases, the characteristic symptoms can include hay fever, skin rashes and asthma. The link between histamine and the blood sugar exists because histamine and glucose are on separate ends of a seesaw. If the glucose level drops, the histamine level rises and vice versa. It follows that a patient who has low blood sugar may, under certain conditions, also have asthma or hay fever.

It is an interesting fact that diabetic patients rarely develop asthma; there are also very few cases on record of an asthma patient also having diabetes. (The main exception is the condition known as cardiac asthma, which is associated with heart disease). Many asthma patients find to their delight in their late 40s and 50s that their asthma symptoms improve. The reason for this is that they are developing late onset diabetes and their blood sugar has become raised above normal level, thus protecting them from asthma.

It should be said that low blood sugar is not the only cause of asthma; there are certain types of asthma caused by stress or extreme sensitivity to various allergens, vigorous exercise, infections and various irritant particles. A good medical dictionary will list more than 30 different types of asthma, usually defined according to their cause.

Musculo-skeletal changes

The other system of the body that is frequently affected by low blood sugar is the musculo-skeletal system – in other words, the muscles and joints. As already explained, the effect of the adrenal glands and, in particular, cortisol on joint inflammation is well documented, hence the apparently miraculous symptom-relief afforded to rheumatoid arthritis patients when cortisol is taken or injected. If the adrenal glands are overworked and fatigued as a result of prolonged low blood sugar, and the efficiency of steroid hormones that protect the joints from inflammation is compromised, joint pain, stiffness and swelling may result. This link between musculo-joint symptoms and stress is known to all of us. The expressions 'pain in the neck' or 'pain in the butt' illustrate the connection. Whether any adrenal exhaustion is caused by stress alone or indirectly caused by low blood sugar, the resulting joint and muscle symptoms are the same.

General symptoms of low blood sugar – the two stages

STAGE ONE SYMPTOMS – FALLING BLOOD SUGAR

The immediate symptoms that follow a fall in blood sugar result from a reduction in the brain and nervous system fuel (i.e. glucose). These first stage symptoms generally include mental and physical lethargy, partial or total loss of concentration, headaches, trembling and/or dizziness, a tendency to yawn, paleness of lips and face with either a skin coldness or heat with perspiration, unexplained anxiety and a sudden urge for chocolate or anything sweet.

STAGE TWO SYMPTOMS – ADRENAL COMPENSATION

The second stage symptoms are caused by the adrenal response to the low blood sugar level. For many people these symptoms are more distressing than those of the first stage.

The surge of adrenaline that occurs in response to low blood sugar causes symptoms identical to the body's response to stress. The metabolism is literally revved up for action. The heart rate increases and the blood flow to muscles is stepped up. This can be likened to pulling out the choke on a car to increase the available fuel. Heavy sweating can occur, with breathlessness and unpleasant palpitations.

A frequent consequence of the stress reaction is a degree of irritability or even aggression – a good example being the mood swings of the diabetic patient. Those readers who have a diabetic friend or relative will know only too well that when a 'hypo' occurs the victim becomes both irritable and aggressive. Many people with low blood sugar symptoms show a degree of anxiety, irritability or depression – symptoms that often improve as their problem is resolved.

All this is part of our body's normal reaction to stress. If we are confronted by an angry bull as we cross a field we need to increase our oxygenation, heart rate and muscle strength to hastily flee. Most athletes and competitive sports people know the value of this adrenaline effect, for the power and speed increase it can provide. They learn to control and at times to override the adrenal response to further their sporting goals.

For most of us this alarm-response by our body is in direct proportion to the intensity of the threat or stress. However, many who suffer with chronic low blood sugar lose their fine control and an adrenal hair-trigger response to stress of any kind leads to frequent and often unnecessary alarm-responses. When adrenaline is released on a regular basis for trivial reasons, many distressing symptoms can develop. Some sufferers, for instance, are frequently awakened at 3–4am bathed in sweat, anxious, with a rapid pulse and short of breath. This occurs because the adrenal response to their nocturnal low blood sugar is being inappropriately triggered and their metabolism is stressed.

Unfortunately, even when we sleep changes in the blood sugar can activate the adrenal response. Professor Hans Selye, who wrote the definitive first description of our response to stress in his landmark 1956 book *The Stress of Life*, described sleep as follows: 'No one is ever absolutely at rest, while alive. Even during sleep, your heart, your respiratory muscles, your brain continue to work. It makes no difference that you are not conscious of this and that these activities require no voluntary effort on your part'.

Our management of stress is a very individual quality that depends on many factors. The amount and type of activity appropriate to a five-year-old child would be very stressful for a 75-year-old man and vice versa. Our stress load and our stress handling are unique to each of us. Stress can, of course, be on many levels, psychological, chemical, structural or environmental. It does not always need to be unpleasant or unexpected to give rise to symptoms. Enjoyable, planned events can also be stressful – excited children becoming sick at parties and sports people suffering asthma attacks are examples of this.

Trigger factors

The most common triggers that can cause low blood sugar symptoms include one or more of the following:

* Excessive sugar consumption.
* Unexpected shock from any cause.
* Unaccustomed or excessive exercise.
* A delayed or missed meal.
* Excessive caffeine intake (e.g. cola drinks or coffee).
* Excessive alcohol.
* The 3- to 5-day pre-menstrual time for women.

CHAPTER 4

The diagnosis of low blood sugar

I have diagnosed and treated patients with low blood sugar for 35 years, and over this time I have learnt that a simple diagnosis of 'low blood sugar' is rarely helpful for the patient and not always accurate. Indeed the diagnostic challenge with low blood sugar symptoms is to provide satisfactory answers to the following questions:

1 Are the symptoms of low blood sugar seen in a patient the result of poor stress handling or a faulty diet, and therefore transient and probably reversible?
   or
2 Are the symptoms the result of a chronic glandular imbalance, long-term stress, excessive reliance on caffeine, tobacco, alcohol and other drugs, or the many other factors associated with dysglycaemia?

In fact, many people with the symptoms of low blood sugar have several causes running parallel. As low blood sugar masquerades as so many different conditions, and can create such a diversity of symptoms, diagnosis can be difficult. For this reason, and others that will be discussed later, it is not wise to diagnose low blood sugar without professional help. Low blood sugar mimics very many serious diseases and it is therefore essential that the possibility of more serious causes for the symptoms is ruled out.

The clinical diagnosis of low blood sugar falls naturally into several stages.

Family history

Low blood sugar disorders can pass from generation to generation. It therefore follows that a detailed evaluation of a person's family health is of considerable diagnostic value.

Table 1 – The family connection, 25 patients

	Condition	Mother	Father	Children	G/Parents	Siblings
PATIENT 1	Migraine	D	–	–	–	–
PATIENT 2	Migraine	–	D	–	D	–
PATIENT 3	Fatigue	M	De	–	–	A
PATIENT 4	Migraine	–	–	H/F	–	D
PATIENT 5	Migraine	–	M	–	D	–
PATIENT 6	Migraine	A+M	–	–	–	A
PATIENT 7	Asthma	–	A	H/F	–	H/F
PATIENT 8	Obesity	F	D	–	–	–
PATIENT 9	Fatigue	M	–	A	–	–
PATIENT 10	Fatigue	M	De	–	–	M
PATIENT 11	Asthma	–	–	–	A	–
PATIENT 12	Obesity	M	D	–	–	O
PATIENT 13	Migraine	–	M	–	–	M
PATIENT 14	Migraine	O	–	H/F	–	A
PATIENT 15	Obesity	M	–	–	D	A
PATIENT 16	Fatigue	D	M	M	–	–
PATIENT 17	Migraine	M	–	–	–	M
PATIENT 18	Depression	–	De	–	–	H/F
PATIENT 19	Hay Fever	D	–	H/F	–	A
PATIENT 20	Obesity	D	–	O	–	O
PATIENT 21	Depression	–	D	F	D	–
PATIENT 22	Fatigue	O	D	–	–	F
PATIENT 23	Migraine	–	–	H/F	–	A
PATIENT 24	Obesity	–	–	–	D	F
PATIENT 25	Fatigue	M	–	H/F	–	–

KEY: *A: Asthma, D: Diabetes, De: Depression, F: Fatigue, H/F: Hay Fever, M: Migraine, O: Obesity*

Table 1 illustrates the family history of 25 patients with confirmed low blood sugar. These patients have been selected because they are typical low blood sugar cases. You will see that characteristic disorders pass through each family. The majority of patients with low blood sugar symptoms tend to show a previous history in their family of either asthma, migraine, hay fever, diabetes, obesity, chronic fatigue or depression.

Present symptoms

As we know, the symptoms of low blood sugar can be misleading to the diagnostician. Often of more significance than a list of symptoms are the pattern of cause and the time of onset of symptoms. One patient, Mr A, may experience headaches when reading or watching television, while another patient, Mr B, may develop headaches only in the early morning or when he drinks certain types of wine. In the case of Mr A, he may well have eyestrain, but Mr B could be suffering from low blood sugar.

Fatigue at the end of the day may be caused by overwork, anaemia or a variety of ailments. Fatigue on rising, which improves towards the end of the day, offers a strong clue to the possible diagnosis of low blood sugar. A subjective evaluation is never easy, for unless one is familiar with the diagnostic value of symptom patterns, it is very difficult to diagnose one's own problems.

One of the chief characteristics of low blood sugar sufferers is the combination of physical and mental symptoms coupled with considerable variation in the symptoms. Sometimes the patient may feel on top of the world; at other times he or she may feel exhausted and depressed for no apparent reason. Remember, we are not dealing with a predictable organic disease such as arthritis or anaemia, but an imbalance in the nervous, circulatory, digestive and endocrine systems. Therefore any symptoms may be the expression of a great number of interrelating and fluctuating causes. These causes can include diet, emotional state, menstruation, time of day, stress, fatigue, the side effects of drugs and many other factors.

Past health

No illness suddenly arrives. There are always changes in the body before the symptoms become apparent to the patient. With low blood sugar the early symptoms are usually vague and difficult to identify. The commonest symptoms are fatigue associated with a dulling of concentration, irritability and mild anxiety or depression, feeling thick-headed on waking and a distinct loss of zest before mid-morning.

Early symptoms may also include transitory feelings of panic or breathlessness with cold sweating and headaches, often accompanied by a craving for something sweet. Such symptoms are often diagnosed as being due to overwork, stress or just 'nerves'. The usual sedatives and relaxants are prescribed, but if symptoms are caused by low blood sugar, any relief will be only temporary. The fatigue will still be there, often without excessive effort or work, and the anxiety will persist, despite a lack of stress.

It is unfortunate that many people with low blood sugar suffer their symptoms because of a false diagnosis. Often they are classified by doctors and family as neurotic when, in fact, the cause of their symptoms is physiological and not psychological.

When looking into a person's history, disorders often feature that provide clues to future low blood sugar. These include hepatitis, jaundice, morning sickness during pregnancy, biliousness and intolerance of fats, a history of gall bladder trouble, chronic fatigue and overweight. The role of the body's early warning system is to indicate the development of a biochemical imbalance or damage of some kind. If the early symptoms of low blood sugar are accurately diagnosed before the obesity, fatigue, migraines and diabetes develop, a great deal of pain and distress may be avoided.

Dietary habits

Faulty nutrition is the single most important cause of low blood sugar. The modern Western diet, with its high sugar content, refined starches, artificial additives and low nutritional value, provides an appropriate formula for causing blood sugar imbalances. If we also consider the modern habits of snack meals, frequent coffees and the excessive use of drugs, alcohol, cola drinks and tobacco, it is no surprise that the incidence of high and low blood sugar conditions is increasing at an alarming rate.

As poor diet is a key factor in the development and maintenance of low blood sugar, it is obviously an important clue in the diagnosis of the problem. I find in practice that most low blood sugar sufferers have characteristic dietary habits that provide important leads to the cause of their symptoms. It must be remembered that, for these patients, meals are not simply a question of choice, for the pattern of meals and type of food is strongly influenced by the underlying low blood sugar. Sugary foods and drinks and caffeine-rich or alcohol-rich drinks all provide temporary relief to the symptoms of low blood sugar. Not surprisingly, the diet reflects this and is usually high in these items and in particular there may be cravings for sweet foods far in excess of normal consumption. One of the most significant clues is a person's sugar intake – two to three teaspoonfuls in either tea of coffee is not unusual. Smoking can also be a clue, as many tobacco addicts experience low blood sugar symptoms.

Because our blood sugar is linked to the appetite, a frequent symptom is hunger. This is not a general feeling of hunger, but more often a craving for a certain type of food. However, the low blood sugar patient, because of the symptoms produced by his condition, often cannot face food. This usually occurs at breakfast time as the blood sugar drops overnight. The thought of breakfast can make a person with low blood sugar feel physically sick. Usually a coffee or cigarette starts the day, and the inevitable 'high' provided by the caffeine produces a mid-morning 'low' as the blood sugar drops again. So the day consists of small frequent 'shots' of sugar or caffeine to maintain the energy level and the concentration at a tolerable level.

When the blood sugar has sunk to a low level, usually around 3–5am, the low blood sugar sufferer often wakes with stomach cramp, indigestion or just hunger – for this reason they are often night nibblers.

The two diets listed below are those of two patients seen in my practice. Every characteristic of the typical eating habits associated with low blood sugar can be seen here.

Example 1
Breakfast: Cereal with sugar and milk, 4–5 cups of tea with 1 teaspoonful of sugar in each cup
11am: Tea with a biscuit or cake
Lunch: Sandwich with tea and biscuit
4pm: Cake with tea
Dinner: Meat and vegetables with sweet dessert, cup of tea
Supper: Crackers, cheese, biscuits and tea

Tea: 12–14 cups daily
Coffee: rarely
Cigarettes: 20–30 a day
Sweets and chocolate: 100–175g (4–6oz) a day
Alcohol: 20–25 units weekly

Example 2
Breakfast: 2 coffees with 2½ teaspoonfuls of sugar in each
11am: Coffee with biscuits
Lunch: Toast with egg or cheese, 2 coffees
4.30pm: Cake with coffee
Dinner: Meat and vegetables followed by coffee
Supper: Cake with coffee

Tea: nil
Coffee: 8–10 cups daily
Cigarettes: 10–12 a day
Sweets and chocolate: 50g (2oz) a day
Alcohol: 15–18 units weekly

Physical examination

There is only one physical sign linked to low blood sugar – a tenderness over the pancreas in the left upper quadrant of the abdomen, often extending as low as the umbilicus. This tenderness is felt just below the ribs, or at times round the side of the ribcage. It is caused by pancreatic sensitivity due to hyperinsulinism. (The functions of the pancreas include the secretion of various substances including insulin to lower blood sugar, and glucogon to raise the blood sugar.) In practice, I find that if I press most patients' abdomens hard enough they are tender in most places. It is important therefore to press with the same gentle pressure all over the stomach, liver and pancreas areas – and then ask the patient, 'which is the most tender?' The fingers encounter a feeling of tightness, or even hardness, accompanying the discomfort. This sign usually disappears as treatment progresses and provides confirmation that the situation is normalizing.

   Although the patient's weight, colouring, blood pressure and so on are all significant in low blood sugar, they are all influenced by many other disorders and are therefore not of special value in diagnosing low blood sugar.

The six-hour glucose tolerance test (GTT)

Often a two to three hour GTT is requested by doctors and hospitals, but although this shortened test may be sufficient for a diagnosis of diabetes, it is virtually valueless as a means of establishing a diagnosis of low blood sugar. The important evidence of low blood sugar can often only occur after more than two hours.

The six-hour GTT test is a far more appropriate method of diagnosing low blood sugar. However, in my opinion it is only a valid diagnostic tool if the following conditions are met:

1   It is combined with a physical examination.
2   A detailed case history is recorded before the test.
3   The patient has described and listed his own diet and symptoms.
4   The patent's reactions and symptoms during the test are noted and timed.
5   The glucose dosage and timing of blood sample taking is standardized for every test.
6   No dramatic changes have recently been made to the diet.
7   The physician is fully aware of any drugs being taken by the patient.

It must be remembered that some people show mild symptoms while other patients show pronounced symptoms even with a 'normal' blood sugar level, hence the need to standardize the test procedures and to know each patient as thoroughly as possible before the test.

TEST PROCEDURE (AUTHOR'S PROTOCOL)

The patient is requested to undergo a 14-hour fast (water only permitted), and to attend the surgery at 9.00am. The fast is no great hardship as only breakfast is missed. Obviously it is important that no food or drink (except water) is taken until the test is completed at 3.30pm. As cigarettes and certain drugs influence the blood sugar it is essential not to smoke during the test, and patients are requested to provide information at least a week before the test on their current medical treatment.

During the course of the test, seven small blood samples are taken. The first sample, taken at 9.15am, shows the level of fasting blood sugar (FBS). At 9.30am the patient is given 50g (2oz) of soluble glucose dissolved in approximately 500ml (16fl oz) of water. The remaining six blood samples are then taken to monitor the effects of the glucose on the patient's blood sugar level. The amount of glucose used in the GTT can vary, 100g (4oz) being the usual test dose in the US. This higher dose can occasionally make the more sensitive patients nauseous or faint, and it is not normally used in the UK. (There is no available evidence to suggest that the higher dose improves diagnostic accuracy.)

The blood sugar level is constantly changing and even with seven samples taken in six hours, one obtains only a guide to the dynamics of blood glucose activities. For this reason, the highest reading may in fact lie between two samples. If I suspect that this has occurred and the speed of the patient's insulin response has been so rapid that the GTT has not confirmed a diagnosis, a repeat test is carried out. This is a shorter version, also using 50g (2oz) of glucose, but with a sample taken every 15 minutes over a $1^{1}/_{2}$-hour period. In this way the all-important upper figure is more precisely assessed.

The timing of when the samples are taken is obviously at the convenience of the practitioner. I find the following schedule most suitable.

Patient arrives		9.00am
Sample 1	FBS taken	9.15am
	50g glucose taken	9.30am
	(drunk quite rapidly with	
	2 glasses of still mineral water)	
Sample 2	–	10.00am
Sample 3	–	10.30am
Sample 4	–	11.30am
Sample 5	–	12.30pm
Sample 6	–	2.00pm
Sample 7	–	3.30pm

This means that the samples are taken after the following amount of time has elapsed since drinking the glucose.

Sample 2	–	½ hour
Sample 3	–	1 hour
Sample 4	–	2 hours
Sample 5	–	3 hours
Sample 6	–	4½ hours
Sample 7	–	6 hours

The patient is encouraged to rest during the test as exercise can influence the blood sugar level, so most patients doze or read. People rarely feel very alert once the test is completed, so it is advisable to arrange to be driven home. It is also sensible to have a small protein snack as soon as possible after completion of the test.

The results of the test usually return from the laboratory within 48 hours but if a glucometer is used the results are available the same day.

SYMPTOMS PRODUCED BY THE GTT

The symptoms that arise during the test and the timing of the onset of these symptoms are both of diagnostic value.

When the glucose readings are explained to the patient on his or her next visit, it is always interesting to note that the symptoms experienced during the test (for example nausea, headache, stomach pains, lethargy, dizziness) usually developed as the blood sugar fell. The majority of patients are impressed to learn that their symptoms – often attributed to stress or their imagination – can be reproduced simply by taking a glucose drink. For them, this confirms the diagnosis of low blood sugar in a far more tangible way than could a set of blood test results. This clinical confirmation of a puzzling condition is often very reassuring to the patient.

Where patients have a long-term condition, however, for example migraine, asthma, fatigue and so on, the symptoms do not always reproduce during the six-hour test.

I have seen GTT results showing profound low blood sugar changes, yet the patient has felt quite well during the testing. This apparent lack of reaction to the changes that occur during the test may be explained in two ways:

1 The patient's metabolism has adjusted to the condition over many years, usually as a result of glandular compensation. Although symptoms still exist, 50g (2oz) of glucose is not sufficient to reproduce these symptoms during the test, although the glucose *is* sufficient to produce the characteristic drop in the blood sugar level.
2 There is frequently a delayed symptom response to the test. For this reason, I always advise patients that they may feel unwell the next day.

GTT RESULTS

The GTT is a valuable test for establishing a diagnosis of diabetes or low blood sugar. Although the orthodox medical view holds that low blood sugar is a rare condition, the evidence points to the contrary. I have found that out of 300 patients selected and tested with a six-hour GTT, 85 per cent showed clearly defined low blood sugar results.

Since Seale Harris first described low blood sugar in 1924, no single generally accepted definition for this condition has been agreed upon. The GTT is open to various interpretations, depending on the doctor's view of what constitutes a 'normal' result. (As with many types of measurement used in medicine, the figures for the average patient cannot necessarily be regarded as the norm.)

Dr Harris has stated that, in his view, a diagnosis of low blood sugar is justified if the GTT shows a blood sugar reading *below* the commonly accepted lower limit of 4mmol/L. This, he insisted, must be supported by the reproduction of low blood sugar symptoms during the course of the test. Over the intervening years, the required lower limit below which low blood sugar could be established and diagnosed has been reduced to 3mmol/L.

This rather rigid criterion for diagnosis has fortunately been modified in recent years, with the general recognition that each GTT result should be assessed in relation to the patient. An individual's response to the glucose drink should be observed in terms of speed of absorption and speed of insulin response. A patient may have pronounced symptoms of low blood sugar yet show a set of glucose readings that are within 'normal' limits. Close attention to symptoms before and during the GTT is of greater diagnostic value than slavish adherence to a set of 'normal ranges'. I have seen patients experience distressing symptoms of low blood sugar when their blood sugar has fallen during a GTT from 8mmol/L to 4mmol/L, the symptoms being caused not by the level of glucose but by the inappropriate speed of the fall.

Let us look at some 'typical' GTT results and the manner in which the result is presented. When the glucose has been taken by the patient, the blood sugar rises (samples 2 and 3). As the glucose is absorbed, insulin is automatically released to control the rising blood sugar. With a normal insulin response, only an optimum amount of insulin is released, allowing the blood sugar level to fall to match the patient's fasting level (sample 7 will therefore show the same level as sample 1).

Normal six-hour GTT result

Sample 1	–	4.4mmol/L
	50g (2oz) glucose taken	
Sample 2	–	6.6 mmol/L
Sample 3	–	5.3 mmol/L
Sample 4	–	4.7 mmol/L
Sample 5	–	4.1 mmol/L
Sample 6	–	4.2 mmol/L
Sample 7	–	4.4 mmol/L

Reactive hypoglycaemia (mild low blood sugar)

Sample 1	–	4.2 mmol/L
	50g (2oz) glucose taken	
Sample 2	–	6.8 mmol/L
Sample 3	–	3.8 mmol/L
Sample 4	–	2.7 mmol/L
Sample 5	–	3.6 mmol/L
Sample 6	–	3.8 mmol/L
Sample 7	–	4.0 mmol/L

Reactive hypoglycaemia (severe low blood sugar)

Sample 1	–	4.5 mmol/L
	50g (2oz) glucose taken	
Sample 2	–	6.2 mmol/L
Sample 3	–	7.4 mmol/L
Sample 4	–	4.6 mmol/L
Sample 5	–	1.8 mmol/L
Sample 6	–	2.1 mmol/L
Sample 7	–	2.8 mmol/L

Flat fatigue GTT (result of adrenal exhaustion)

Sample 1	–	4.7 mmol/L
	50g (2oz) glucose taken	
Sample 2	–	4.8 mmol/L
Sample 3	–	4.8 mmol/L
Sample 4	–	5.2 mmol/L
Sample 5	–	4.5 mmol/L
Sample 6	–	4.7 mmol/L
Sample 7	–	4.7 mmol/L

Diagnosis using the GTT

When presented with a set of figures for a GTT, the first step for the diagnostician is to look for a possible diabetic component. A fasting level in excess of 8mmol/L is strongly suggestive of diabetes, but some diabetics can have a fasting level under 6mmol/L. For this reason an assessment of the sum of the first four results obtained in the GTT is a more reliable method of identifying diabetes. If the total for the four samples is between 28–44mmol/L, diabetes is suspected; if it is over 44mmol/L, diabetes is positively confirmed.

There are many different types of GTT results, for the dynamics of the blood sugar level are expressed in many ways. It is very unusual to find any two GTT curves that are alike, so it is important to bear in mind that so-called 'normal' values are based on population averages and may not reflect what is normal for the patient being tested.

The actual level of blood sugar is related to symptoms during the test, but even more important, perhaps, is the speed at which the blood sugar responds to the insulin. A drop from 6.5mmol/L to 3.5mmol/L in one hour may be more significant than a drop from 6.5mmol/L to 2.5mmol/L in two hours. The time taken for the sugar to return to a normal level (usually referred to as 'recovery'), and how long it remains at a low level, are also important diagnostic clues. For example, a fall to 2.5mmol/L with a rapid recovery to normal may be less significant than a fall to 3.5mmol/L that stays at this level for two to three hours before recovery.

Some disagreement surrounds the value of interpreting the 'fall' in blood sugar during the test. This represents the difference between the initial fasting level and the lowest figure to which the blood sugar drops during the test. I find in practice that a fall as little as 0.5mmol/L can be associated with low blood sugar symptoms. In the view of Carlton Fredericks, an authority on many aspects of blood sugar, no practitioner should disregard a blood sugar reading that is 'only a few points below normal' and if there is doubt, a diagnosis of low blood sugar with correct treatment should be considered.

Other tests for low blood sugar

Although the six-hour GTT is recognized as the definitive test to identify low blood sugar, the results do not answer the question of what is causing the condition. In an attempt to clearly understand the background cause or causes of low blood sugar, various tests are diagnostically useful. It is not within the scope of this book to delve too deeply into laboratory testing, but a brief description of the most frequently requested tests may interest readers.

Blood insulin measurement

Given how widespread blood sugar problems are, you may understandably assume that checking the insulin level of sufferers is a routine test. Unfortunately this is not so. Although widely used in the US, it is still a relatively rare test in Europe.

Elevated blood insulin (hyperinsulinaemia) is a major component in many syndromes and disorders, including Syndrome X, insulin resistance, PCOS, stage II (late onset) diabetes, low blood sugar and obesity. Not surprisingly, the concept of hyperinsulinaemia has been closely linked to the low blood sugar syndrome for more than 70 years. I frequently request a blood insulin test and raised levels are not unusual.

ADRENOCORTEX STRESS PROFILE

With this test, which can be done at home, two adrenal hormones are measured in a patient's saliva four times over a 24-hour period. Although it is a home saliva test, and the laboratory provides a useful commentary and reference ranges, interpretation requires practitioner experience.

The hormones measured are cortisol (hydrocortisone) and DHEA (dehydroepiandrosterone). These hormones are involved in many important body functions, including protein, fat and carbohydrate metabolism, stress management, inflammation and pain control, and blood sugar balancing. An excess or a deficiency of either of these two hormones can contribute to illness. Low levels have been observed in chronic fatigue disorders, muscle-joint pain and stiffness, stress, anxiety, low blood pressure and low blood sugar.

It is important that cortisol and DHEA are in the correct balance with each other. (Significantly, the blood DHEA falls as the insulin rises. Raised levels of DHEA play a part in protecting against obesity, diabetes and low blood sugar.)

THYROID HORMONE TESTING

The adrenal glands and the thyroid gland functions are closely linked. An imbalance or a deficiency in one gland can influence the other. Hypothyroidism (an underactive thyroid) is known to render the adrenals less efficient and, as we now know, one of the many symptoms caused by adrenal exhaustion or reduced activity is low blood sugar. Conversely, a malfunctioning adrenal system can depress our metabolism and lower thyroid hormone activity. I frequently find that in patients with low blood sugar, both glands are inefficient and a vicious circle of hypofunction has been established. This is shown in the representation overleaf.

The adrenal-thyroid circle

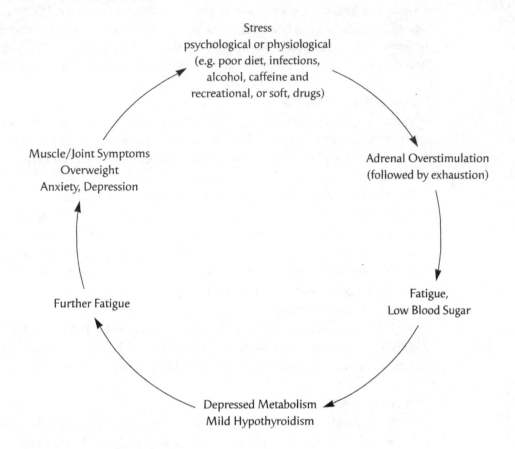

Stress
psychological or physiological
(e.g. poor diet, infections,
alcohol, caffeine and
recreational, or soft, drugs)

Adrenal Overstimulation
(followed by exhaustion)

Fatigue,
Low Blood Sugar

Depressed Metabolism
Mild Hypothyroidism

Further Fatigue

Muscle/Joint Symptoms
Overweight
Anxiety, Depression

The tests

The two main tests included in a thyroid profile are as follows:

* FREE T4 (THYROXINE)
  This is the most valuable test for recognizing a *mildly* underactive thyroid. Many patients are within the laboratory reference range, but their results fall into the lower section of the range and they experience the symptoms of mild hypothyroidism.

* T.S.H. (THYROID STIMULATING HORMONE)
  This pituitary hormone, by definition, is raised to support an underactive thyroid. However, with many people, the pituitary may also be depressed and may fail to recognize a mild hypothyroid. Although the T.S.H. is seen in the UK as the definitive test for thyroid malfunction, in many cases the hormone only increases with severe hypothyroidism and a mildly reduced thyroid output can easily be missed, unless the Free T4 is also requested. For this reason, the symptom-picture and the laboratory findings should always be closely compared. This guideline applies to both thyroid and adrenal function. Glands can be inefficient without being diseased or damaged.

PART TWO

Treating Low Blood Sugar

CHAPTER 5

The low blood sugar diet

There is no one diet recommended by all the various 'experts' for treating low blood sugar. There are, however, certain essential guidelines or requirements that must be met if a diet for low blood sugar is to be effective.

Dietary requirements for a low blood sugar diet

1 Total carbohydrate consumption must be minimal and refined (quickly absorbed) carbohydrates, including sugar, chocolate, sweets and so on, must be avoided.
2 There should be five or six small snack meals daily, with a protein or fat component included in each meal.
3 The total calorie content of the diet should be around 2000–2500 calories. Those who are overweight may need to reduce this to 1200–1500 calories.
4 The diet must include a substantial breakfast and supper, to be taken as early and as late as possible.
5 Stimulants that will increase but subsequently lower the blood sugar (owing to hyperinsulinaemia) must be avoided. These include alcohol, tobacco, chocolate, caffeine and cola drinks.

The various diets on offer for treating low blood sugar are all quite different, yet in each case the diet seems to work – and evidence is available to confirm the efficiency of each regime. The success of these regimes is probably due to certain common factors, namely the avoidance of refined starch and the insistence upon five or six regular meals each day.

However, diets work only if the patient is prepared to follow them for a prescribed period of time. With the low blood sugar diet, it is essential to maintain the diet for an initial period of eight to twelve weeks. This will allow time for your system to adjust to the changes in your diet and to obtain a more stable blood sugar level and subsequent symptom relief.

General requirements for the low blood sugar diet

In formulating the diet, I have tried to take into account the various constraints that many people are subject to, such as budget and a lack of time. I therefore employed the following criteria:

1 It should not contain expensive or exotic food (for example, fillet steak or smoked salmon daily).
2 Many people work full-time and cannot prepare elaborate dishes, therefore the meals must be simple – particularly as there are four to six 'meals' per day to prepare.
3 The diet should not be too unsociable or too different from average meals. Otherwise, I have found that patients are too easily tempted to stray off the recommended foods.
4 The meals should be tasty and enjoyable.
5 Since many low blood sugar sufferers are overweight, and conscious of extra pounds, the diet should not result in weight gain.
6 Finally, and perhaps most obvious, the diet must work. Only by feeling better will someone continue to follow a strict diet, week after week.

Although I frequently draw up individual diets for patients, they are usually based on a standard diet.

Recommended diets for low blood sugar

The standard diet that I use is set out below. This diet is for those who eat meat; on pages 38–40 and 41–3 you will find low blood sugar diets for vegetarians and vegans respectively.

STANDARD LOW BLOOD SUGAR DIET

ON RISING

1 medium orange, ½ grapefruit or 100ml (4fl oz) fresh fruit juice diluted with 50 per cent water, or a cup of decaffeinated coffee or tea, herb or fruit infusions, milk or yogurt

BREAKFAST

Fruit or 100ml (4fl oz) fruit juice
1 egg, with or without 2 slices of ham or bacon, or cheese or fish
1 slice of wholemeal (whole-wheat) bread or toast, with plenty of butter
Milk or other beverage

2 HOURS AFTER BREAKFAST

100ml (4fl oz) fresh fruit juice or, if necessary, a high protein drink

LUNCH
Meat, fish, cheese or eggs with salad (a large serving of lettuce or tomato with
    mayonnaise or French dressing)
Vegetables as desired
Slice of wholemeal (whole-wheat) bread, toast or crispbread with plenty of butter

2 HOURS AFTER LUNCH
100ml (4fl oz) milk or, if necessary, a more substantial high protein drink or snack

1 HOUR BEFORE DINNER
100ml (4fl oz) fruit juice

DINNER
Home-made soup, if desired (not thickened with flour)
Meat, fish or poultry
Vegetables
Slice of wholemeal (whole-wheat) bread, if desired
Dessert of fruit – fresh, stewed or baked
Beverage

EVERY 2 HOURS UNTIL BEDTIME
Small handful of unsalted nuts

SUPPER (AS LATE AS POSSIBLE)
High protein snack i.e. crispbread with cottage cheese or pate, with butter
Milk or other beverage

Notes
Live traditional yogurt made from sheep or goats' milk and containing Lactobacillus
Acidophilus is preferred to synthetic cows' milk yogurt.

Where butter is mentioned, vegetable margarine may be substituted. If dairy
products are unacceptable, owing to catarrh, migraine, asthma or intolerance,
substitute soya milk, plant milk or other non-animal products.

Allowable food and drink
PROTEIN AND FAT SOURCES
Butter, cream, vegetable (or soya) margarine, vegetable oils, cheese, yogurt and milk
(goats', sheep and soya is preferable to cows' milk), meat, poultry, game, fish (fresh and
canned), pulses and lentils, nuts and seeds, tofu.

VEGETABLES

Asparagus, beetroot (beets), broccoli, Brussels sprouts, lettuce, mushrooms, cabbage, cauliflower, carrots, celery, sweetcorn, cucumber, beans, onions, peas, radishes, peppers, aubergines (eggplants), courgettes (zucchini), tomatoes, turnips, swede, parsnips and any other fresh vegetables (potatoes, however, should be eaten only in moderation and with a source of protein for the initial period of the diet). Frozen vegetables and vegetables canned without sugar or salt.

FRUIT

Apples, apricots, strawberries, raspberries, blackberries, grapefruit, melons, oranges, peaches, pears, pineapple, tangerines, avocados and any other fresh fruit. May be cooked or raw with or without cream, but *without* sugar. Avoid canned fruit unless it is sugar free. Eat grapes, plums, figs, dates and bananas and dried fruit only in moderation and preferably with a source of protein (this is not necessary after your blood sugar has stabilized and you are on a 'maintenance' diet).

JUICE

Any unsweetened fruit or vegetable juice, except grape juice or prune juice. Avoid canned fruit or vegetable juice unless pure and sugar free.

BEVERAGES

Decaffeinated coffee or tea, or weak China or Indian tea (occasionally), herb or fruit infusions.

DESSERTS

Fruit – fresh, stewed or baked without added sugar.
Cheese and sugar-free natural desserts.

SALT

Use sea salt in moderation or low sodium salt.

Avoid absolutely

Any foods not mentioned on the diet and, in particular, sugar; chocolate and other carbohydrates such as cakes, pies, pastries, sweet custards, puddings, commercially-made ice cream; salted nuts; all refined cereal products; diabetic foods; syrup, molasses and honey; ordinary coffee, strong tea and other beverages containing caffeine; tobacco; alcohol and soft drinks. It is also advisable to avoid the use of synthetic sugars (see page 37).

WHY THE LOW BLOOD SUGAR DIET

When the majority of patients first encounter the diet prescribed for low blood sugar, they are understandably baffled by the ban on sugar. They have been given a diagnosis of low blood sugar and yet they must avoid sugar. Low blood sugar is the opposite of diabetes and diabetics cannot have sugar, so surely the low blood sugar sufferer must eat lots of sugar?

Throughout our lives we are informed and persuaded that sugar gives us energy. Sugar, honey, glucose and molasses are names synonymous with vitality. The low blood sugar patient is exhausted and depressed. It can, therefore, be very confusing for the low blood sugar sufferer to be told that they will feel better if they avoid all the sugar-rich foods and drinks that are traditionally thought to provide energy.

However, there are sound physiological reasons why sugar and refined carbohydrates must be avoided. Neat sugar is absorbed quickly and the body reacts by discharging insulin into the blood. We know that hyperinsulinaemia is the central problem in our blood sugar and sugar aggravates and perpetuates this problem. Our digestive systems need a small amount of carbohydrate in order to efficiently break down and absorb proteins and fats. This, however, can be supplied by taking non-refined carbohydrates (for example, wholemeal bread, whole-wheat cereal and pasta, and fruit and vegetables) that offer better nutrient value, a higher fibre content and a more gradual conversion to sugar in the blood.

In the context of blood sugar balance, the colour of the sugar is irrelevant. Both brown and white sugar have the same disturbing effects. Honey's sweetness is derived chiefly from sucrose (white sugar) and molasses has similar effects. For this reason both items are barred from the diet.

Synthetic sugars

This is an appropriate point at which to mention synthetic sugars. It is advisable to avoid the use of synthetic sugars. Although, from the purely chemical viewpoint, they should not influence the insulin-glucose balance, there are two facts worth noting:

1 If one needs to follow a low blood sugar diet for several months, and possibly always avoid sweet foods, it makes dieting considerably easier if all forms of sweetness in food are avoided, including synthetic sweeteners (for example, saccharine).
2 Research has shown that synthetic sweeteners trigger the pancreas into activity rather like a conditioned reflux. Even the smell of food can stimulate the gall bladder into activity and many physical changes (allergies, migraine, etc.) can be triggered by the smell and taste of food.

FREQUENCY OF MEALS

An important characteristic of the low blood sugar diet is the need for frequent meals. As we know, the low blood sugar patient produces too much insulin in response to certain foods and, as a result, the blood sugar falls. The only way to avoid a severe drop in the blood sugar is to eat small meals at frequent intervals. Frequent snack meals of starch (sandwiches, cereal, etc.) would serve only to aggravate the problem, as all forms of carbohydrate are absorbed more quickly than proteins and fats. The relatively slow absorption of proteins and fats does not trigger the sensitive insulin response, hence eating snacks containing protein and/or fat ensures that the blood sugar remains stable and sudden rises and falls in the glucose levels are avoided.

This levelling off of the blood sugar throughout the day is extremely important, as it is the *speed* of elevation that triggers off the insulin response and not the *amount* of rise (e.g. an increase of 4–6mmol/L of sugar in the blood will produce a similar pancreatic response as a rise from 10–12mmol/L). The drinks between meals prevent overeating as these serve to reduce the almost unbearable craving for food so characteristic of low blood sugar. The milk drinks do the job of 'topping up' between meals – without them the blood sugar would drop and symptoms would develop. In severe cases it may even be necessary to chew protein tablets between meals or take frequent soya-based protein drinks.

PROTEINS AND FATS

I find the concept of a high-protein or high-fat diet unacceptable and unnecessary, and prefer to talk in terms of a 'protein-fat spread' diet. In simple terms this means that a normal amount of protein and fat is consumed, with plenty of variety in choice of sources, but the fat or protein is eaten at least four times daily. As I have already said, proteins and fats are absorbed slowly and do not severely disturb the insulin-glucose ratio.

Many foods rich in fats (for instance, cheese, yogurt and butter) are recommended in the diet as they serve to depress pancreatic activity. It should be remembered, however, that this diet is a short-term corrective programme, and it may not be appropriate to consume the quantity of fat recommended in the diet for long periods. This particularly applies to patients with a history of obesity or heart or circulation problems, or with a high level of fat in the blood. (It is usual, if a high cholesterol or triglyceride factor is suspected, to measure these with blood tests before placing the patient on the raised fat diet). Although the selection of fats and oils is partly a matter of taste, both are calorie-rich groups so moderation is essential, even with a low blood sugar diet.

In this context it is worth looking at the use of oils to replace solid fats in cooking. The Mediterranean diet, with its emphasis on fowl, fish, oil and garlic combined with fresh fruit and vegetables, offers an ideal basis for an effective diet for the treatment of low blood sugar, without running the risk of increasing the blood fats.

VEGETARIAN DIET FOR LOW BLOOD SUGAR

ON RISING
1 piece of fruit or 100ml (4fl oz) fresh fruit juice diluted with 50 per cent water

BREAKFAST
Fruit or 100ml (4fl oz) fruit juice
Choose one of the following:
Sugar-free baked beans on toast with mushrooms or tomatoes

Vegetarian pate or cheese on toast
An egg dish
Wholegrain cereal with milk
Yogurt with fresh fruit
Drink: Decaffeinated tea or coffee, herbal or fruit teas

2 HOURS AFTER BREAKFAST
100ml (4fl oz) fresh fruit juice or, if necessary, a high protein drink

LUNCH
Mixed fresh salad with French dressing, cider vinegar, lemon juice or sugar-free
    mayonnaise. Add vegetarian savoury rice, cheese, nuts or fruit as desired or eggs.
Slice of wholemeal (whole-wheat) bread or Ryvita with vegetable margarine.
Drink: As breakfast

2 HOURS AFTER LUNCH
100ml (4fl oz) milk or, if necessary, a more substantial high protein drink or snack

1 HOUR BEFORE DINNER
100ml (4fl oz) fruit juice

DINNER
Home-made soup
Mixed vegetables with vegetarian savoury, can include cheese dish, stuffed peppers or
    tomatoes, savoury rice, mushrooms, vegetable pie or casserole, vegetarian savouries,
    lentil savouries, soya dishes, wholegrain pasta or an egg dish.
Dessert of stewed, baked or fresh fruit or yogurt or Ryvita with cheese.
Drink: As breakfast

EVERY 2 HOURS UNTIL BEDTIME
Small handful of unsalted nuts

SUPPER (AS LATE AS POSSIBLE)
A protein snack is essential i.e. vegetarian pate or cheese with Ryvita or bread
Milk or other beverage to drink

Notes
Lunch and dinner may be reversed.

Allowable food and drink

PROTEIN AND FAT SOURCES

Butter, cream, vegetable (or soya) margarine, vegetable oils, cheese, yogurt and milk (goats', sheep and soya is preferable to cows' milk), pulses and lentils, nuts and seeds, tofu. Also don't forget wholegrain cereals, especially high protein ones such as quinoa.

VEGETABLES

Asparagus, beetroot (beets), broccoli, Brussels sprouts, lettuce, mushrooms, cabbage, sauerkraut, cauliflower, carrots, celery, sweetcorn, cucumber, beans, onions, peas, radishes, peppers, aubergines (eggplants), courgettes (zucchini), tomatoes, turnips, swede, parsnips and any other fresh vegetables (potatoes, however, should be eaten only in moderation and with a source of protein for the initial period of the diet). Frozen vegetables and vegetables canned without sugar or salt.

FRUIT

Apples, apricots, avocados, berries, grapefruit, melons, oranges, peaches, pears, pineapple, tangerines and any other fresh fruit. May be cooked or eaten raw, *without* sugar. Avoid canned fruit unless it is sugar free. Eat grapes, plums, figs, dates and bananas and dried fruit only in moderation and preferably with a source of protein (this is not necessary after your blood sugar has stabilized and you are on a 'maintenance' diet).

JUICE

Any unsweetened fruit or vegetable juice, except grape juice or prune juice. Avoid canned fruit or vegetable juice unless it is sugar free.

BEVERAGES

Any natural coffee substitute or decaffeinated coffee and decaffeinated tea. Herb or fruit teas or the occasional weak China and Indian tea.

DESSERTS

Fruit – fresh, stewed or baked without added sugar
Cheese
Sugar-free natural desserts or yogurt

SALT

Use sea salt in moderation or low sodium salt.

Avoid absolutely

Any foods not mentioned on the diet, particularly sugar; chocolate and other sweets such as cakes, pies, pastries, sweet custards, puddings, commercially-made ice cream; salted nuts; refined cereals; diabetic foods; syrup, molasses and honey; ordinary coffee, strong tea and other beverages containing caffeine; tobacco; alcohol and soft drinks. It is also advisable to avoid the use of synthetic sugars (see page 37).

PLANT PROTEINS

The basic components from which proteins are made are amino acids. There are eight amino acids that cannot be synthesised by our metabolism and must therefore be present in the food we eat. These essential or indispensable amino acids are isoleucine, leucine, lysine, methionine, phenylalanine, threonine, tryptophan and valine.

Unfortunately, although animal proteins (with the exception of gelatine) contain all the essential amino acids, vegetable proteins lack one or more. However, with a varied diet the amino acids in one food can complement those in another. This means that a vegan diet for low blood sugar *can* work but a variety of vegetables, seeds, nuts and fruits are necessary.

VEGAN DIET FOR LOW BLOOD SUGAR

ON RISING
1 piece of fresh fruit or 100ml (4fl oz) fresh fruit juice diluted with 50 per cent water

BREAKFAST
Fruit or 100ml (4fl oz) fruit juice
Choose one of the following:
Sugar-free baked beans on toast with mushrooms or tomatoes
Vegetarian pate or vegan cheese on toast
Wholegrain cereal with soya milk
Drink: Herb tea, decaffeinated coffee, weak China or Indian tea

2 HOURS AFTER BREAKFAST
100ml (4fl oz) fresh fruit juice or, if necessary, a high protein drink

LUNCH
Mixed fresh salad with French dressing, cider vinegar, lemon juice or sugar-free
    mayonnaise. Add vegan savoury, rice, vegan cheese, nuts or fruit as desired.
Slice of wholegrain bread or Ryvita with vegetable margarine.
Drink: As breakfast

2 HOURS AFTER LUNCH
100ml (4fl oz) fruit juice or, if necessary, a more substantial high protein drink or snack

1 HOUR BEFORE DINNER
100ml (4fl oz) fruit juice

DINNER
Home-made soup or fruit
Mixed vegetables with vegan savoury i.e. vegan cheese dish, stuffed peppers or
    tomatoes, savoury rice, vegetable casserole, lentil savouries, or soya dishes.
Desserts: Stewed, baked or fresh fruit
Drink: As breakfast

EVERY 2 HOURS UNTIL BEDTIME
Small handful of unsalted nuts

SUPPER (AS LATE AS POSSIBLE)
A protein snack is essential i.e. vegan pate or cheese or soya milk with Ryvita or bread.

Notes
Lunch and dinner may be reversed.

Allowable food and drink
PROTEIN AND FAT SOURCES
Vegetable (or soya) margarine, vegetable oils, vegan cheese, soya milk and yogurt,
pulses and lentils, nuts and seeds, tofu. Wholegrain cereals, especially high protein
ones such as quinoa.

VEGETABLES
Asparagus, beetroot (beets), broccoli, Brussels sprouts, lettuce, mushrooms, cabbage,
sauerkraut, cauliflower, carrots, celery, sweetcorn, cucumber, beans, onions, peas,
radishes, pepper, aubergines (eggplants), courgettes (zucchini), tomatoes, turnips,
swede, parsnips and any other vegetables (potatoes, however, should be eaten only in
moderation and with a source of protein for the initial period of the diet). Frozen
vegetables and vegetables canned without sugar or salt.

FRUIT
Apples, apricots, berries, grapefruit, melons, oranges, peaches, pears, pineapple,
tangerines, avocados and any other fresh fruit. May be cooked or eaten raw, *without*
sugar. Avoid canned fruit unless it is sugar free. Eat grapes, plums, figs, dates and
bananas and dried fruit only in moderation and preferably with a source of protein
(this is not necessary after your blood sugar has stabilized and you are on a
'maintenance' diet).

JUICE
Any unsweetened fruit or vegetable juice, except grape juice. Avoid canned fruit or
vegetable juice unless sugar free.

BEVERAGES
Any natural coffee substitute or decaffeinated coffee. Herb or fruit teas or the occasional weak China or Indian tea.

DESSERTS
Fruit – fresh, stewed or baked without added sugar.
Vegan cheese and sugar-free natural desserts.

SALT
Use sea salt or low sodium salt in moderation.

Avoid absolutely

Any foods not mentioned on the diet, particularly sugar; chocolate and other sweets such as cakes, pies, pastries, sweet custards, puddings, commercially-made ice cream; salted nuts; refined cereals; diabetic foods; syrup, molasses and honey; ordinary coffee, strong tea and other beverages containing caffeine; tobacco, alcohol and soft drinks. It is also advisable to avoid the use of synthetic sugars (see page 37).

THE NIGHT-TIME FAST

The low blood sugar diet requires that the patient has an early breakfast and a late supper. Both these meals should include either fat or protein. This recommendation is made to reduce the hours one spends 'fasting' throughout the night. As has been discussed in preceding chapters, the blood sugar normally falls to a low level between the hours of 3–5am. The early morning asthma attack, the onset of migraine, panic feelings and anxiety, night-time raids on the kitchen and so on are all expressions of this phenomenon. By reducing the hours between dinner and breakfast, these symptoms can be improved or eliminated. The majority of people eat their last meal around 7pm and have breakfast at 7am. This 12-hour 'fast' is too long, and careful, regular eating throughout the day is pointless if a patient develops a low blood sugar episode every night.

I advise patients to eat a small protein supper prior to going to bed (10.30pm– midnight) and to have a glass of milk on waking (6.30–7.30am). If, in spite of this, the severe early morning symptoms persist, I have at times recommended that patients set their alarm for around 3am and have a small meal at this time. This may be tedious, but, if the early morning symptoms can be suppressed for four to six weeks, it can be considered to be well worthwhile. After such a time the diet and other measures have usually normalized the insulin-glucose balance sufficiently to allow the patient to sleep through the night.

Prolonged fasting

Patients often ask the question, 'If fasting aggravates low blood sugar, causing distressing symptoms, why is it that patients in health clinics can fast for five to 10 days and yet feel marvellous?' The answer to this is in two parts. Firstly, they do not feel 'marvellous' – at least not during the first two days. Patients undergoing a fluid-only fast almost certainly experience many symptoms of low blood sugar. These include headaches, irritability, nausea, dizziness and indigestion. (A true low blood sugar patient would, of course, experience more profound and sustained symptoms.) Secondly, prolonged fasting does not cause a severe, progressive fall in the blood sugar. This is prevented by the process known as 'endogenous catabolism', which simply means that the body breaks down and utilizes its own fat and protein reserves. Patients who are literally starving to death with various forms of cancer, often show no symptoms of low blood sugar, the average blood sugar of patients tested being 4.5–5mmol/L. This compensation process that occurs during fasting only begins to operate after the third or fourth day of the fast, hence the initial drop in blood sugar during the first 48 hours of the fast.

Tea, coffee, alcohol, cola drinks and smoking

All these substances, directly or indirectly, contribute to the low blood sugar condition and must, therefore, be eliminated from the diet. It is particularly important to avoid the above list during the first few weeks of the diet, when the insulin response is still very sensitive. Patients whose low blood sugar has been controlled by the proper diet can show severe blood sugar reactions when they take as little as *one* cup of coffee. Many investigators have shown that exposure to a smoky atmosphere (passive smoking) can be virtually as harmful as smoking. For this reason the low blood sugar patient should avoid restaurants, theatres, parties etc. where the atmosphere is smoky.

CHAPTER 6

The Glycaemic Index

In 1995, when I described the Glycaemic Index (GI) in the book *Recipes For Health –
Low Blood Sugar* (published by Thorsons), the GI was a relatively new concept. It is used
to measure the rate of carbohydrate food absorption, which has relevance to changes in
the blood sugar levels.

HOW THE GLYCAEMIC INDEX IS MEASURED
The standard measuring method for the many hundreds of different foods is relatively
straightforward. Volunteers are given specific portions of food and their blood sugar is
then measured and compared with their response to glucose. The carbohydrate content
of each food tested is previously worked out using food composition tables. The blood
sugar response to individual foods is then compared with an equivalent of glucose and
the GI of each food is established.

The factor, or GI, of foods affects the speed of conversion of foods to blood sugar
(glucose). High value foods show a rapid response and subsequent increase in the blood
sugar (for example, glucose has a GI of 100). Conversely, complex carbohydrates and
low GI range foods (e.g. those below 50) are absorbed slowly, causing a gradual rise in
the blood sugar. Using this standard measuring method, the GI of many hundreds of
different foods is now known.

You may at this point ask 'yes, but what is the GI of meals that can contain eight to
ten different food items?' The GI value of a complete meal can be assessed if the carbohydrate content of each food eaten plus the total carbohydrate content of the entire meal
is known. The blood sugar response can then be measured and a 'meal GI' provided.

WHY DOES THE GI OF FOODS VARY?
Many factors influence the GI of foods. These include starch content, fibre content, fat
content, sugar content and the food processing and cooking methods used.
Accompanying foods and drinks can also influence the total meal GI (e.g. the use of
acidic salad dressings, vinegar and fruit juices).

The value of selecting foods with a low GI lies in the speed of their conversion to
glucose in the blood. Foods with a low GI convert to glucose more slowly than foods with

a high GI. Therefore a diet rich in low GI foods requires less insulin to bring the blood sugar under control. Unfortunately, although such a diet will consist largely of low sugar foods, the actual nutritional value of foods (i.e. their vitamin and/or mineral content) is not a factor when considering the GI of foods for meal and menu planning. The GI is a useful guide when selecting foods for a low blood sugar diet, but low GI foods are not necessarily healthy food – ice cream, for instance, has the same GI as yogurt.

However, foods with a low GI are appropriate for inclusion in an effective diet to treat low blood sugar. It can be safely stated that the lower GI foods are better than the high GI foods when it comes to designing a low blood sugar diet.

THE GLYCAEMIC INDEX OF SOME COMMON FOODS

SUGARS	GI	VEGETABLES	GI
Fructose	22	Beetroot	64
Glucose	100	Carrot	92
Honey	87	Fresh Peas	33
Sucrose	65	Frozen Peas	51
		Mashed Potato	50
CEREAL PRODUCTS	GI	Potato	70
All Bran	51	Parsnips	97
Brown Rice	68		
Cornflakes	80	PULSES	GI
Oatmeal Cereal	49	Baked Beans	40
Shredded Wheat	67	Kidney Beans	29
Spaghetti	50	Lentils	29
Sweetcorn	59	Lima Beans	36
Swiss Muesli	66	Soya Beans	15
White Bread	62		
White Rice	72	DAIRY PRODUCTS	GI
Whole-grain Bread	72	Ice Cream	36
		Skimmed Milk	32
FRUIT	GI	Whole Milk	34
Apple	39	Yogurt (plain)	36
Apple Juice	45		
Banana	62	VARIOUS	GI
Orange	40	Chips (French Fries)	75
Orange Juice	46	Chocolate Bar	68–76
Raisins	64	Coca Cola	63
		Peanuts	13
		Pizza (average)	62
		Potato Crisps	51
		Soya Milk	32

CHAPTER 7

Case histories

The cases featured in this section are all those of real patients. However, readers should not assume that because the symptoms discussed sound like their own that the treatments suggested are suitable for them. There is no such person as a typical patient. We are all very different and any diagnosis, diet and supplements prescribed can vary according to the individual being treated.

Case history – Pam

SYMPTOMS

Pam, a 35-year-old teacher, had experienced many symptoms of low blood sugar since puberty. Her ongoing symptoms included fatigue with poor short-term memory and concentration. The fatigue was at its worst on waking, something that wasn't helped by her habit of waking between 3–4am most mornings with a powerful appetite, which she satisfied by bingeing on biscuits and sweet drinks.

Perhaps not surprisingly Pam was overweight. She weighed 73kg (11st 7lb or 161lb), which, with a height of 158cm (5ft 2in), gave Pam a body mass index, or BMI, of 29 – this isn't quite into the 'obese' range but is at least 13kg (28lb) overweight. (An ideal BMI weight at her height is 49–64kg (7st 10lb–10st or 108–41lb).

Pam claimed to 'never feel warm' and suffered with almost daily frontal headaches and rhinitis. She experienced sugar cravings, weight increase and moodiness for six to seven days before her period. Pam's libido was non-existent and she was unmarried.

The family history provided significant diagnostic clues. Pam's father and mother both suffered from chronic migraine, her mother's mother had been a diabetic and her mother's sister suffered hypothyroidism. In addition, Pam's two brothers both experienced seasonal hay fever.

Pam's diet featured a great deal of carbohydrate foods, such as sandwiches and pasta, and very little protein. (Such a diet usually results from a combination of cost-cutting and sugar cravings). She drank 6–8 cups of coffee and 5–6 units of alcohol daily and smoked 15–20 cigarettes daily.

Having consulted many therapists and tried different diets over a period of 20 years, without lasting success, she was desperate for some 'facts and figures' and a more precise diagnosis to explain her symptoms.

DIAGNOSIS

I requested a six-hour GTT, coupled with a general blood screen – including a thyroid profile. The GTT showed a normal fasting glucose but three of the tests showed results under 3mmol/L. In addition to this confirmation of low blood sugar, Pam's tests also indicated a mild hypothyroidism. Her work was a source of stress, particularly as her fatigue and poor memory added to the workload. The symptoms of adrenal exhaustion, so often cross-linked with low blood sugar and mild hypothyroidism, contributed to Pam's fatigue, poor stress handling and PMS.

TREATMENT

I prescribed a low carbohydrate diet with frequent protein-rich snacks (see pages 141–54), coupled with nutritional, glandular, thyroid and adrenal support, and a specific glucose tolerance supplement (see Glossary). I also recommended soluble potassium to treat her low blood sugar levels, and omega-6 (Evening Primrose Oil) to counteract her PMS.

After four months, Pam was feeling a little better, especially on rising. The vicious circle of fatigue, stress and yet more fatigue was beginning to break up and her optimism and self-confidence were improving. She is still very overweight but, with her gradual thyroid improvement and the reduction in the bingeing and sugar cravings that were caused by her low blood sugar, any future weight-loss programmes should work more speedily and permanently.

Case history – Simon

SYMPTOMS

Aside from the occasional menopause patient in her late 40s or early 50s, the majority of my low blood sugar patients are less than 40 years old. Simon, at 55 years, was an unusual patient for several reasons. He described himself as an 'intermittent alcoholic'. He was very overweight, with widespread joint pain and muscular stiffness. His other symptoms included mood swings, anxiety and very poor short-term memory and concentration. He also had an abnormal thirst and dry hair. However, his low blood sugar symptoms, which included morning fatigue, snacking between meals and chocolate cravings, had only been with him for three years.

Simon's doctor had advised him to reduce his alcohol as a health priority (his intake being approximately 10–15 units each day). Fortunately, he had taken the advice and had been 'dry' for the previous six months when he came to see me. His weight was 90kg (14st 2lbs or 198lbs), which, with a height of 173cm (5ft 8in), gave him a BMI of

30 – just into the obese range. He also had high blood pressure and high blood tri-glycerides (blood fat) and a depressed HDL cholesterol (the so-called 'good' cholesterol).

As a self-employed accountant, Simon was a sedentary desk worker.

DIAGNOSIS

Simon's symptom cluster pointed to a possible diagnosis of insulin resistance, raised blood insulin and Syndrome X (see page 8). I therefore requested a fasting blood insulin test and a test to measure the essential fatty acids (omega-3 and omega-6). I also requested a DHEA measurement – DHEA in the blood usually falls when the blood insulin rises.

The results confirmed the likely diagnosis of Syndrome X, the low blood sugar symptoms being part of the syndrome, not the cause. Simon's tests showed low omega-3 levels, a reduced DHEA and an elevated blood insulin. To add confirmation to the diagnostic jigsaw puzzle, Simon's father was a late onset diabetic and his mother had hypothyroid obesity.

TREATMENT

The priority with Syndrome X is to reduce the sugar and calorie content of the diet. Simon was advised to also reduce his intake of saturated fats in favour of fish and fish oils. He was prescribed the G.T.F. Complex™ (see page 165), supplementary omega-3, the protein Carnitine, Vitamins C and E, and DHEA.

With a gradual reduction in his weight, Simon's blood fats and blood pressure gradually normalized over a 10-month period. During this time his weight reduced by 13kg (28lb) to a weight of 77kgs (12st 2lb or 180lb), giving him a BMI of 26. This weight loss has encouraged him to be more active – he now enjoys walking and swimming – and his increased vitality has lead to an improvement in his memory and concentration. The combination of improved adrenal efficiency and exercise also reduced Simon's chronic muscle and joint stiffness.

Case history – Jennie

SYMPTOMS

Jennie, a 32-year-old newspaper reporter, had been self-treating her low blood sugar since the age of 12. Her mother had treated her own low blood symptoms for most of her life, but neither had been entirely successful in obtaining symptom-relief.

Prior to reading my first book on low blood sugar, a year earlier, Jennie had been experiencing severe morning headaches with fatigue, poor concentration and short-term memory, anxiety, mood swings and severe PMS. She found most people irritating and, given her occupation, her symptoms were causing her work to suffer.

As stress of any type can contribute to low blood sugar symptoms, a vicious circle of stress, symptoms and more stress can be established. This was happening with Jennie and her strategy of simply reducing sugar, coffee and chocolate was not sufficient to break the circle and provide symptom relief. There was clearly more to do and when Jennie contacted me she was only feeling slight relief after changing her diet.

With many early-stage health problems such as PMS, diabetes, gout, candidiasis and low blood sugar, dietary intervention can lead to a dramatic improvement. However, with chronic problems that can continue for years, a variety of secondary problems and symptoms can develop – examples being excess weight, high blood pressure, poor stress handling, poor immunity, low libido, mineral and vitamin deficiencies and, perhaps the most commonly seen symptoms of any chronic health problem, fatigue.

DIAGNOSIS

It was obvious Jennie suffered many symptoms of low blood sugar. However, her symptoms had been with her since puberty and 20 years of ill health were not going to be completely reversed by simply removing chocolate, coffee and sugar from her diet.

As Jennie's mother was experiencing virtually the same symptoms, an inherited mineral deficiency seemed possible. I therefore requested a Serum Mineral Profile. The minerals tested include calcium, magnesium, zinc, copper, iron, manganese and chromium. The chromium level in Jennie's blood particularly interested me. The mineral chromium is a chief component of the 'glucose tolerance factor' molecule, which assists insulin-glucose metabolism. In the words of Dr Robert C. Atkins, 'chromium is far and away the most pivotal nutrient involved in sugar metabolism'. He also asserts that 'more than 90 per cent of all Americans are deficient' in this nutrient.

Unfortunately, much of the soil in the West is chromium deficient and excessive sugar in the diet can further deplete our chromium stores. Jennie's blood showed low levels of magnesium, manganese, zinc and chromium.

TREATMENT

I encouraged Jennie to tighten up her diet with the addition of protein drinks every hour between meals and prescribed soluble potassium (Sando-K) on rising (see page 164). I also prescribed my G.T.F. Complex™ (see page 165), which contains, amongst many other things, magnesium, manganese, calcium, potassium, zinc, vanadium and chromium.

After six months, Jennie was almost free of her symptoms. She still experienced mild mood swings and sugar cravings prior to her periods, but her general vitality was much improved. With the return of her physical vitality she also improved mentally. Her moodiness, forgetfulness and concentration lapses gradually cleared.

Case history – Adam

SYMPTOMS

Adam's morning temperature averaged 35.6°C (96°F), yet he regularly awakened at around 3–4 am with heavy night sweats. (The normal waking temperature, when taken under the arm for 10 minutes, is 36.6–36.8°C [97.8–98.2°F]).

He was a 24-year-old office worker suffering from chronic fatigue (which was much worse before lunch), anxiety, depression, indigestion and very poor immunity and stress-handling. These symptoms had been with him for nine years. However, the morning fatigue and night sweats had persisted since early childhood. When he consulted me he had been off work for six months and had been diagnosed as suffering stress-induced gastritis, with anxiety and depression. Anti-depressant drugs had been prescribed and counselling was also recommended.

Adam admitted to being a 'fussy eater' and his very poor diet confirmed this, consisting mainly of refined carbohydrates and little in the way of protein and fats.

Adam's diet

BREAKFAST 7–8AM
Cereal with milk and sugar
White toast with marmalade
2–3 cups of coffee with sugar

LUNCH 1–2PM
Sandwiches with cheese or marmite (2 rounds)
2–3 cups coffee with sugar

AFTERNOON SNACK 4–4.30PM
Cake or biscuits, 1 cup of coffee with sugar

DINNER 7–7.30PM
Usually chicken breast or beefburger
Chips and baked beans
1–2 small beers

SUPPER
Packet of crisps, 1 coffee with sugar

As is obvious from the above list, Adam rarely ate fruit, salad or fish. He drank 6–8 cups of coffee and 3–4 units of alcohol daily and smoked 10–15 cigarettes daily.

In her excellent book *Let's Get Well*, Adelle Davis states that 'During severe stress as much as 135gms of body protein [the amount in 600g or 1¼lb of lean steak or 20 medium eggs] may be destroyed in a single day'. Many who believe they are eating a high protein diet, with an egg for breakfast and meat for dinner, are only obtaining around 25 grams or one ounce of protein each day. This can be easily remedied by taking high protein drinks.

Adam's habit of waking in the early hours of the morning is common. Patients frequently ask why they tend to waken around 3–4am with feelings of panic and stress. Normal adrenal gland function peaks in the early hours and falls to the lowest point at midnight. The role of the adrenal gland is to raise the blood sugar between 3–4am by releasing cortisol (hydrocortisone). This hormone stimulates the liver to release glycogen (glucose stores). If a patient's blood sugar falls too rapidly or falls below the normal level the resulting 'hypo' will trigger an excessive adrenal response that can cause palpitations and anxiety, coupled with excessive sweating in the waking patient. If the adrenal response to the nocturnal fall in blood sugar is not efficient, a person will wake up feeling tired, irritable and anxious as a direct result of the delayed adrenal surge.

DIAGNOSIS

I requested that Adam have an Adrenocortex Stress Profile (saliva samples) and the results showed a low morning cortisol (hydrocortisone) and a low noon cortisol. His DHEA was also below the reference range. All this pointed to adrenal hypofunction with resulting low blood sugar symptoms.

TREATMENT

I prescribed my usual low blood sugar diet and in addition advised Adam to have a protein drink mid-morning, mid-afternoon and mid-evening. These drinks are an easy and inexpensive way of increasing protein intake. For additional support, and to ease his night sweats, I advised him to set his alarm clock for 2.30am and to have a protein drink and snack meal at this time. He was routinely awakened by palpitations and sweating, so his sleep pattern was not further disturbed.

I prescribed my G.T.F. Complex™, 50mgs of DHEA daily and the Adreno-Lyph Plus for nutritional adrenal support. In addition, I recommended that Adam take one Sando-K (soluble potassium – see page 164) on waking and one on retiring, for a period of six weeks.

Within three months, the adrenal support and extra protein began to reduce his symptoms and after eight months of treatment Adam was virtually symptom-free. He discontinued his night snack after four months and he now sleeps through the night without the heavy sweating, consequently he feels much more refreshed upon waking.

Case history – Peter
SYMPTOMS

When Peter's wife made his first appointment she explained to my secretary that he had only agreed to see me to please his family. He considered that his mood swings, aggressive tendencies and excessive drinking were all symptoms of his high-pressure work.

Peter, a 40-year-old record producer, described himself as an 'adrenaline freak'. I later discovered that his wife was on the point of leaving him but, with two children and many mutual supportive friends, she had decided to first seek a few answers. She wanted to know if Peter was suffering from a personality disorder or was the victim of a hidden health problem.

At his consultation, I found him to be a slim, pleasant person with a deceptively relaxed manner. He had a very good diet and did not drink coffee, eat sweets or chocolate, or smoke. He did, however, drink around 10 units of red wine each day. After a little persuasion he admitted that he was at times forgetful. His physical symptoms included fatigue on rising, chronic throat infections, and stomach bloating after meals, coupled with heartburn. He also suffered from frequent mouth ulcers and laryngitis 2–3 times each year.

Peter had been diagnosed as hypothyroid five years earlier and was currently taking 125mcgms of thyroxine daily. His family history revealed a diabetic father, and a sister and mother who were both thyroid cases. Although Peter's symptoms were threatening his marriage, he really could not see 'what all the fuss was about'.

Those with low blood sugar symptoms, which can include morning lethargy, moodiness and aggression, often fail to understand the effects that their symptoms can have on their family and friends. Falls in the blood sugar can lead to a defensive, petulant attitude in the victim. This was well demonstrated with Peter. (Other typical examples of the effects of low blood sugar on personality can be seen in alcoholics and women with PMS.)

DIAGNOSIS

Peter had read widely on low blood sugar and he considered that his very good diet and his sugar, coffee and tobacco avoidance were the only 'treatments' needed. His justification for his alcohol habit – he drank the equivalent of two bottles of wine each day – was that it was necessary to help him relax. He believed the wine was preferable and safer than taking drugs for anxiety.

I considered it possible that his fluctuating blood sugar and stressful lifestyle had rendered his adrenals inefficient and his thyroid activity had also been depleted. I therefore requested a thyroid profile (ensuring that Peter took his thyroxine at least 12 hours before the blood test).

In the UK, patients tested for the thyroid hormone Free T4 (thyroxine) are given the same reference range whether they are taking thyroxine or not. In the US and Australia, and many other countries, those patients on thyroxine (i.e. over 100mcgms each day) are given a higher reference range to allow for the thyroxine effect. However, when the reference range is not adjusted for the thyroxine dosage a 'normal' result can be given when hypothyroid symptoms are still present. Peter's Free T4 result was 10.6pmol/L. With a normal reference range of 8–19pmol/L, Peter was therefore declared 'normal and stable'. In fact, when allowing for his thyroxine dosage of 125mcgms, an appropriate reference range should be 20–30pmol/L (assuming symptom-relief). To further understand something of Peter's adrenal system I requested a saliva Adrenocortex Stress Profile (see Glossary). This showed a low cortisol (hydrocortisone) and a low DHEA activity. This type of result, showing reduced adrenal hormone levels, is typically found in those suffering chronic stress, fatigue and low blood sugar. A diagnosis of adrenal fatigue, or exhaustion, is often used to describe this phenomenon.

TREATMENT

Although Peter followed a healthy diet, it was not an ideal diet for treating low blood sugar. When treating blood sugar disorders, whether low blood sugar or diabetes, the timing of meals is of great importance. A late protein or fat-based supper and an early breakfast are both essential. Long gaps between meals are not appropriate. I therefore advised Peter to follow the frequent-meal pattern of my standard low blood sugar diet. Many patients can experience typical low blood sugar symptoms within two hours of eating. To counteract this I often recommend high protein soya drinks between meals with a protein or fat component in each meal.

I prescribed a nutritional thyroid support (Thyro-Complex) for Peter and an adrenal glandular supplement (Adreno-Lyph Plus). I also recommended the G.T.F. Complex™ to provide the B-complex vitamins and the essential minerals for blood sugar metabolism. In addition, I advised Peter to take soluble potassium chloride. Potassium is lost in the urine with stress, resulting in sodium (salt) and fluid being retained. When this urinary loss of potassium is replaced with 1–2gms of potassium, the blood sugar generally increases. I usually recommend Sando-K (available over the counter at any pharmacist), which contains 600mg of potassium chloride and 400mg of potassium bicarbonate in each soluble tablet. Potassium supplements are available in health stores but the dosage is usually only 200–300mgs. (Potassium supplements should not be taken where there is a history of kidney disease or by those who are following low potassium diets). Peter was advised to take one tablet on rising in fruit juice to help to reduce his morning low blood sugar symptoms.

After four months of treatment, Peter was less moody and more in control of his symptoms. His wife was reassured that his symptoms were largely physiological not psychological. Unfortunately when domestic and business stress contributes to the low blood sugar symptoms, progress can be slow and rarely 100 per cent. An ideal diet is always good therapy. However, there are times when selected specific nutritional supplements are also necessary.

Case history – Katy
SYMPTOMS

Before new patients see me for a consultation they must first complete a questionnaire on their family history, medical history, current symptoms, and any prescription drugs or supplements they may be taking. They must also include a three-day diary of their food and drink intake, including information on tea, coffee, alcohol, cola drinks, tobacco and sugar use, in addition to the precise timing of meals. The benefits of having such data prior to seeing a patient are obvious and time-consuming questions can be minimized.

Katy's form was puzzling. She was a 19-year-old, symptom-free student with no medical history, a perfect diet and no bad eating or drinking habits. My trepidation was confirmed when, upon meeting Katy, she stated 'I don't know why I am here'. Katy was nearing the end of her first year at university, where she was taking a three-year degree course. She was achieving very good grades and was very happy with the course. Unfortunately her parents had heard a different story, via a family friend who was on the faculty. He had heard from colleagues that Katy's behaviour at the college was causing some concern.

Katy's mother had listed their comments, which were that Katy was increasingly irritable, at times irrational, unfocused and 'spaced out'. Her time-keeping was very poor, she was sleeping during lectures and showed an aggressive attitude and behaviour. Perhaps most significant, was the statement that Katy 'seemed unaware and indifferent to other students' impressions of her'. Although these were typical low blood sugar symptoms, there was no obvious cause. Furthermore, Katy's mother had failed to notice any changes in her daughter's behaviour during her holidays at home.

However, it emerged that the three-day diary that Katy had sent to me described her eating habits at home. I therefore requested details of her food and drink at university. Her behavioural changes had gradually developed 3–4 weeks into her first term.

Katy's university diet

BREAKFAST
Cereal with milk and sugar, 2 coffees with 2 teaspoons of sugar per cup

10–10.30AM
Coffee and biscuits

LUNCH
Sandwich, coke, chocolate bar, crisps, plus 2 coffees

4–4.30PM
2 coffees, crisps or biscuits

6.00PM
Pasta or chips, crisps and 2 coffees

10–10.30PM
Biscuits and 2 coffees

Katy rarely ate fruit, salads or vegetables. She did not drink alcohol or smoke. However, she ate peppermints throughout the day. Her daily sugar consumption included 30–35 teaspoons of sugar, biscuits, chocolate bars, sweets, cereals, crisps and pasta. Virtually the only protein she ate was a little meat sauce with her pasta, and ham or cheese with her lunchtime sandwich.

TREATMENT

When questioned it became quite clear that Katy had no interest in food and failed to see any link between her behaviour and her eating habits. With her mother's help I persuaded her that her diet was very poor and could eventually make her ill. I gave her a copy of my book *Low Blood Sugar* to provide the 'evidence'. She agreed to a 'change-of-diet' trial for one term. In addition to providing Katy with a diet plan, I also gave her information on protein-rich drink recipes to take between meals. I also stressed the importance of potassium-rich fruits (for instance, dried apricots, dried peaches, figs etc.) and strongly advised her to reduce her sugar habit. The G.T.F. Complex™ was prescribed to ensure the essential minerals and vitamins were in Katy's daily diet.

After the trial term, the reports on Katy's behaviour were very encouraging. Although she had originally complained at the unnecessary attention from her parents and friends, she admitted she was feeling generally more vital and relaxed.

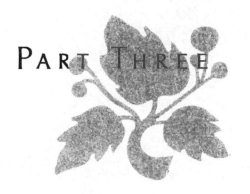

Part Three

The Recipes

Chapter 8

Introduction

The essential guidelines for a successful diet to treat low blood sugar have been listed in Part Two. However, a reminder of the essence of the diet and the timing of meals is appropriate before we delve into the recipes.

A unique feature of a diet for low blood sugar is the need to eat frequently, hence five to six snacks and/or meals each day are often required. While this may sound like a lot of food – and a lot of fuss – it actually fits in well with most peoples' routines and eating habits. The days of the family all eating together at mealtimes seem to be long gone, as does a strict adherence to the traditional three meals a day. These days, pressure of time and work mean it's more common for breakfast and lunch to be solitary affairs, with families only getting together for the occasional shared dinner. While this is not necessarily a positive thing for the family, it does make life simple for those following a low blood sugar diet. It means you can prepare your own particular breakfast and lunch – be it at home or to take to the office – and in the evening enjoy a meal that all the family can share, if they want.

The drinks and small snack meals that are part and parcel of the plan are also easily incorporated into the daily routine. Most of us tend to have a snack mid-morning and mid-afternoon – so we simply need to adhere to the ban on sugary foods and drinks and instead enjoy a simple unsweetened fruit juice or high protein snack. Having had a substantial breakfast, many people find a fruit juice mid-morning is enough to stabilize their blood sugar until lunchtime; while others will need something a little more substantial. The mid-afternoon and evening snacks are also important as there is often a long period between lunch and dinner, dinner and supper. The only other requirement regarding snacks is to have one before going to bed – hardly a chore! As food avoidance can cause low blood sugar, a late supper serves to reduce the 'on-waking' symptoms so characteristic of low blood sugar.

Whilst eating frequently and enjoying decent breakfasts and late snacks may seem like a recipe for weight gain, fortunately the required avoidance of high sugar foods and drinks usually ensures a reasonably low total daily calorie count – an important factor as many of those with low blood sugar also have weight problems.

BREAKFASTS

We all tend to avoid food for eight to 10 hours through the night, and the unfortunate modern habit of missing breakfast and instead having a snack at around 11am only makes matters worse – lengthening the night fast to as much as 12 to 15 hours. However, for anyone suffering the symptoms of low blood sugar, breakfast is the most important meal of the day. In the past, when more people were involved in manual labour, workers knew the value of breaking the night fast with a substantial meal that included meat, fish, eggs or cheese. Unfortunately, many 21st-century workers rely instead on sugary snacks and drinks to keep them going through the morning.

This is a particularly bad strategy for those with low blood sugar, who require a substantial protein-rich breakfast to raise their blood sugar and keep it stable. In practical terms this means that you simply must eat breakfast – no excuses. You can have wholemeal toast or sugar-free cereal but your breakfast must also include protein-rich food. Prolonged food avoidance causes low blood sugar levels and those who suffer poor blood sugar control learn to dread waking – so reverse the trend and have a good breakfast as early as possible.

LUNCH AND DINNER

When planning a diet to treat low blood sugar, the main meals do not require the change of mindset that is necessary when thinking of appropriate snacks. This is because the main guidelines of the diet – to exclude sugary foods and include protein in meals – are easily applied to these meals. Most of us automatically include a protein component in our lunch and dinner. However, we tend to choose the same protein sources – for instance, dairy produce, chicken and red meat. Variety is important in a healthy diet so if they're not already a part of your diet introduce fish (fresh and canned), game, pulses, tofu and nuts.

Salads are a popular choice for packed lunches, as well as side dishes for dinner and main courses in the summer. They are an important part of a healthy diet – but do remember to add protein (plant or animal) and/or a fat constituent if you are serving salad as a main meal.

BETWEEN-MEALS SNACKS AND DRINKS

Many who read this book will have experienced the symptoms of low blood sugar as a result of food avoidance. The dizziness, mood changes, fatigue and headaches that are symptomatic of low blood sugar can develop within just two hours of eating. For this reason, between-meals drinks and snacks are a crucial part of the diet.

Unfortunately, many people equate the word snack with sweet cakes, sugary biscuits or cookies, and chocolate – all things that negatively affect the blood sugar. In contrast, the recipes for snacks that follow will help to keep your blood sugar on an even keel – and they are also easy to prepare, tasty and convenient. Remember, snacks do not have to be sweet – sugar-free natural yogurt, hard-boiled eggs, crackers and cheese, or a handful of unsalted nuts, all provide ideal between-meal nibbles for preventing blood sugar slumps.

One of the easiest and most important snacks are protein drinks – these are a great low-cost source of protein and are particularly good as a supper snack as they ensure you feel more refreshed on waking. Some soya-based drinks can taste rather bland to some palates so, if you wish, add some sugar-free juice for extra flavour – try, for instance, prune, blackcurrant or pineapple (a non-citrus juice is best).

FOOD QUALITY

The quality of the food we eat directly affects our health, so to get the best out of your diet it is vital to eat the best quality food you can afford. Choosing organic food is the best means of avoiding all the harmful chemicals that foods – be they animal or vegetable – are subjected to. Thankfully, all types of organic foods are now becoming much more readily available – fresh fruit, vegetables, cheeses, fish, fowl, game and meat can all now be bought from various sources. Supermarkets are stocking more and more organic produce (and if you cannot visit the store you can always shop online) but other important sources include the numerous farmers' markets now in existence and the specialist suppliers who will deliver organic produce direct to your door. In some areas, it also now possible for local communities to buy produce direct from co-operatives of local farmers. (See Resources for a list of suppliers).

Organic produce may seem expensive to those on a limited budget but remember, if you cut out all the sweet and refined foods from your diet, you will be saving money in the process. Sugar-rich, refined convenience foods are not only expensive in terms of money – they take a heavy toll on our health.

Beating low blood sugar for life

The recipes in this section are designed to fit in with the plan outlined on page 34, however they are also appropriate for inclusion in a long-term maintenance diet. Once your blood sugar has stabilized, it is essential not to return to a high sugar diet as this would only result in a recurrence of symptoms. Although it is unnecessary to stick to *all* the rules of the diet for life, to experience continued relief from symptoms it is necessary to continue to avoid sugary foods and drinks and carbohydrate-only meals as much as possible, and to eat at regular intervals. Though this may at present seem troublesome and restrictive, once you have achieved symptom relief it will become a routine part of your regular healthy diet. Do continue to use the recipes in this section as part of that maintenance plan – they are delicious, energy giving and full of flavour. Even those that you may find a little 'unusual' to begin with will soon become favourites – yes, to this day we still love sardines for breakfast!

CHAPTER 9

Breakfasts

High Protein Cereal

Ingredients

METRIC (IMPERIAL)		AMERICAN
100g (4oz)	soya flour	1½ cups
175g (6oz)	rolled oats	¾ cup
2 tablespoons	bran	2 tablespoons
3 tablespoons	wheatgerm	3 tablespoons
125ml (4fl oz)	vegetable oil	½ cup
25g (1oz)	sesame seeds, toasted	¼ cup
25g (1oz)	sunflower seeds, toasted	¼ cup
100g (4oz)	raisins	⅔ cup

Method

1 Preheat the oven to 170°C/325°F/gas mark 3.

2 Mix all the ingredients except the sesame seeds, sunflower seeds and raisins.

3 Spread the mixture on a non-stick baking tray. Roast for 35–45 minutes, stirring occasionally.

4 Allow the mixture to cool then add the remaining ingredients.

5 Store in an airtight container.

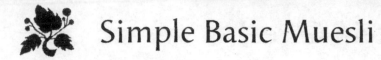

Simple Basic Muesli

Ingredients

METRIC (IMPERIAL)		AMERICAN
50g (2oz)	barley flakes	1¼ cups
50g (2oz)	rye flakes	1¼ cups
100g (4oz)	oat flakes	1 cup
50g (2oz)	wheat flakes	1¼ cups
50g (2oz)	raisins	⅓ cup
100g (4oz)	rolled oats	1 cup
50g (2oz)	mixed nuts, coarsely chopped	½ cup
50g (2oz)	sunflower seeds	⅓ cup
1 large	eating apple	1 large

Method

1 Mix all the ingredients in a large bowl.

2 Grate some apple into each serving just before eating.

Note

Any fresh fruit can be added to replace the apple, or chopped dry fruit. The oats can be soaked overnight in water for ease of digestion.

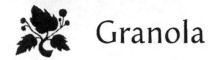

Granola

Ingredients

METRIC (IMPERIAL)		AMERICAN
450g (1lb)	oat flakes	1lb
3 tablespoons	sunflower oil	3 tablespoons
50g (2oz)	sesame seeds	⅓ cup
50g (2oz)	desiccated (shredded) coconut	⅔ cup
50g (2oz)	hazelnuts, chopped	½ cup
few drops of	pure vanilla extract	few drops of
100g (4oz)	raisins	⅔ cup

Method

1 Preheat oven to 190°C/375°F/gas mark 5.

2 Mix all the ingredients, except the raisins, in a large bowl.

3 Spread the mixture on a baking tray and cook for 20–25 minutes. Turn the mixture regularly to ensure even roasting.

4 When golden brown, remove from the oven and allow to cool.

5 When completely cold, stir in the raisins.

6 Store in an airtight container.

Beans and Cheese on Toast

Few of us have time to make our own sugar-free baked beans, so the canned variety are a good convenience food for all those who lead busy lives.

Ingredients

METRIC (IMPERIAL)		AMERICAN
1–2 slices	wholemeal (whole-wheat) bread	1–2 slices
200g (7oz)	Heinz sugar-free baked beans	1 cup
75g (3oz)	mature Cheddar cheese, grated	¾ cup
	freshly ground black pepper	

Method

1 Toast the bread on one side only. Set aside.
2 Meanwhile, heat the beans thoroughly then mix in the cheese.
3 Season with pepper, spread over the untoasted side of the bread and grill (broil) until bubbling.

Sardines on Toast

Ingredients

METRIC (IMPERIAL)		AMERICAN
4	canned sardine fillets in olive oil, drained	4
100g (4oz)	butter	½ cup
	lemon juice	
	salt and freshly ground black pepper	
2–3 slices	wholemeal (whole-wheat) bread	2–3 slices

Method

1 Place the sardines and butter in a small mixing bowl and mash together until thoroughly mixed.

2 Add a squeeze of lemon juice and season with salt and pepper.

3 Toast the bread on one side. Spread the sardine mixture on the untoasted side and grill (broil) for 4–5 minutes until brown.

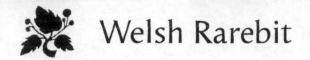

Welsh Rarebit

Ingredients

METRIC (IMPERIAL)		AMERICAN
4 slices	wholemeal (whole-wheat) bread	4 slices
100g (4oz)	mature Cheddar or Red Leicester cheese, grated	1 cup
1 teaspoon	mustard powder	1 teaspoon
1 teaspoon	Worcestershire sauce	1 teaspoon
pinch	paprika	pinch

Method

1 Toast the bread on one side only.
2 Place the remaining ingredients in a mixing bowl and mix well together. Spread the mixture over the untoasted sides of the bread.
3 Grill (broil) for 3–4 minutes until the cheese browns.

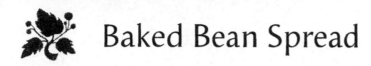

Baked Bean Spread

This spread can also be used as a sandwich or baked potato filling.

Ingredients

METRIC (IMPERIAL)		AMERICAN
200g (7oz) can	Heinz sugar-free baked beans	1 cup
	freshly ground black pepper	
75g (3oz)	low-fat Cheddar cheese, grated	¾ cup

Method

1 Put the baked beans in a mixing bowl, mash well and season with pepper.

2 Add the cheese and mix thoroughly.

3 Use as a sandwich filling, or toast the bread on one side and spread on the mixture, then grill (broil) until brown and bubbling.

4 Store any leftover spread in a covered bowl in the fridge and eat the following day.

CHAPTER 10

Lunchtime snacks and sandwiches

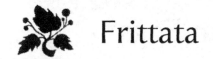

Frittata

This simple egg dish is also known as a flat omelette or tortilla. It can contain any variety of vegetables and cheeses. This dish could become a mainstay for those who take a packed lunch to work. A slice of cold frittata plus a nutritious salad will provide a substantial lunch.

Ingredients

SERVES 4

METRIC (IMPERIAL)		AMERICAN
2 tablespoons	olive oil	2 tablespoons
1 large	red onion, thinly sliced	1 large
3	courgettes (zucchini), cut into matchsticks	3
	salt and freshly ground black pepper	
5 medium	eggs, lightly beaten	5 medium
75g (3oz)	feta cheese, cubed	1 cup
2 tablespoons	fresh basil, chopped	2 tablespoons

Method

1 Preheat the grill (broiler) on a high heat.
2 Heat half the oil in a medium non-stick frying pan (skillet) and cook the onion until soft and lightly browned.
3 Add the courgettes (zucchini) and plenty of seasoning and continue cooking until golden.
4 Combine the eggs, cheese and basil and season well.
5 Remove the onion and courgette (zucchini) mixture from the pan with a slotted spoon and add to the egg mixture, mixing well.
6 Wipe the pan clean and heat the remaining oil. Add the egg mixture and cook over a low heat, stirring occasionally, until partially set but not brown.
7 Place the pan under the preheated hot grill (broiler) to cook the top of the frittata. Do not allow the frittata to stay for long under the grill (broiler) as it will dry out.
8 Serve warm or cold, cut into wedges.

Variations

Other possible ingredients include pumpkin, broccoli florets, red (bell) pepper, potato (cubed or finely sliced), sun-dried or fresh tomatoes, baby leeks, asparagus, garlic, young green beans, fresh goat's cheese, Parmesan cheese and fresh herbs – especially parsley and thyme.

Anchovy and Parmesan Eggs

Ingredients

METRIC (IMPERIAL)		AMERICAN
8	anchovy fillets, drained	8
4 large	eggs	4 large
	freshly ground black pepper	
50g (2oz)	unsalted butter	¼ cup
2 tablespoons	Parmesan cheese, grated	2 tablespoons

Method

1   Chop the anchovies. Lightly beat the eggs and season with a little pepper.

2   Melt half the butter in a saucepan, reduce the heat and pour in the eggs.

3   With the eggs still slightly liquid, stir in the remaining butter with the cheese and the anchovies.

4   Serve on thinly sliced hot buttered wholemeal (whole-wheat) toast.

Tomatoes Stuffed with Cottage Cheese and Tuna

Ingredients

METRIC (IMPERIAL)		AMERICAN
4	slicing (beefsteak) tomatoes, very ripe	4
150g (5oz)	canned tuna in oil, drained and flaked	¾ cup
1	anchovy fillet, chopped	1
1 teaspoon	capers, chopped	1 teaspoon
150g (5oz)	cottage cheese	¾ cup
bunch	fresh parsley, chopped	bunch

Method

1 Cut the tomatoes in half, remove the seeds and most of the pulp. Discard the seeds and reserve the pulp. Season the tomatoes with a little salt.

2 In a mixing bowl, combine the tuna, anchovy fillet, capers, reserved tomato pulp, cottage cheese and most of the parsley.

3 Stuff the tomatoes with the mixture, sprinkle with the remaining parsley and serve with a mixed green salad.

Cream Cheese, Celery and Anchovy Ciabatta Rolls

Ingredients

METRIC (IMPERIAL)		AMERICAN
10	anchovy fillets in oil, drained and chopped	10
50g (2oz)	cream cheese or Quark	¼ cup
1	small celery stick, thinly sliced	1
	freshly ground black pepper	
	butter or soya margarine for spreading	
2	wholemeal (whole-wheat) ciabatta rolls	2
	crisp lettuce, finely shredded	

Method

1 Mix together the chopped anchovy, cheese, celery and pepper.
2 Butter the rolls and spread the mixture on both halves of the rolls. Fill with the lettuce.

Variation
You could spread a thin smear of Gentleman's Relish (Patum Peperium) on the rolls as an alternative.

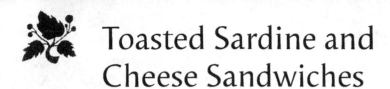

Toasted Sardine and Cheese Sandwiches

These sandwiches also make a tasty breakfast dish.

Ingredients

METRIC (IMPERIAL)		AMERICAN
4	canned sardine fillets	4
50g (2oz)	cream cheese or Quark	¼ cup
	salt and freshly ground black pepper	
8 slices	wholemeal (whole-wheat) or granary bread	8 slices
8–10	crisp lettuce leaves	8–10

Method

1 Drain the sardines, chop well and place in a mixing bowl.
2 Add the cheese and seasoning and stir until thoroughly combined.
3 Spread the mixture over all 8 slices of bread.
4 Place the lettuce over 4 slices then place the remaining 4 slices on top, sardine-side down.
5 Toast on both sides under a preheated hot grill (broiler).

Note
The sardines should be canned in olive oil.

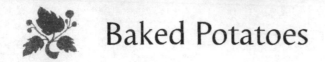

Baked Potatoes

Ingredients

METRIC (IMPERIAL)		AMERICAN
1 large	baking potato (King Edward, marfone etc.)	1 large

Fillings

bacon, cooked until crisp and cut into
  small pieces
Cheddar cheese, grated
smoked tofu, thinly sliced
baked beans (sugar-free)
fromage frais with chopped chives

mixed salad to serve

Method

1　Preheat the oven to 200°C/400°F/gas mark 6.
2　Cut round the potato, just cutting into the skin.
3　Bake in the preheated oven for 1–2 hours, depending on size. Alternatively, cook in the microwave on full power for 10–20 minutes until nearly cooked and then finish in the oven to give the skin a nice crispy finish.
4　Serve with your choice of filling and a bowl of mixed salad.

Sardine, Egg and Watercress Sandwich

Ingredients

METRIC (IMPERIAL)		AMERICAN
4	canned sardines, drained and coarsely chopped	4
1 large	egg, hard-boiled and chopped	1 large
1 tablespoon	mayonnaise	1 tablespoon
2 teaspoons	lemon juice	2 teaspoons
	salt and freshly ground black pepper	
4 slices	wholemeal (whole-wheat) bread	4 slices
	butter or soya margarine for spreading	
handful	watercress, chopped	handful

Method

1 Place the sardines and egg in a mixing bowl. Add the mayonnaise, lemon juice and seasoning and mix well.

2 Butter the bread, fill with the sardine mixture, top with watercress and sandwich together.

Herb and Mushroom Sandwich

Ingredients

METRIC (IMPERIAL)		AMERICAN
2 tablespoons	olive oil	2 tablespoons
1	small onion, finely chopped	1
175g (6oz)	open-capped mushrooms, finely chopped	2¼ cups
1 tablespoon	fresh parsley, chopped	1 tablespoon
2 teaspoons	lemon juice	2 teaspoons
25g (1oz)	peanuts, chopped	2 tablespoons
	salt and freshly ground black pepper	
4 slices	wholemeal (whole-wheat) bread	4 slices
	butter or soya margarine for spreading	
	lettuce leaves, shredded	

Method

1 Heat the oil in a frying pan (skillet) and cook the onion for 3–4 minutes, until nearly soft.

2 Stir in the mushrooms and continue cooking for 5–6 minutes.

3 Mix in the parsley and lemon juice, bring to the boil then simmer until most of the liquid has evaporated. Stir in the peanuts.

4 Leave to go cold then season to taste.

5 Butter the bread, fill with the mushroom mixture, top with the lettuce and sandwich together.

Croque Campagnard

Ingredients

METRIC (IMPERIAL)		AMERICAN
1 thick slice	country bread such as ciabatta, pain de campagne or any rustic wholemeal (whole-wheat) bread	1 thick slice
	butter for spreading	
1 thin slice	ham (Parma or Bayonne)	1 thin slice
25g (1oz)	Gruyere (Swiss) cheese, grated	¼ cup

Method

1 Toast the bread very lightly on both sides.

2 Lightly butter the toast, cover with the ham and sprinkle with cheese.

3 Cook under a preheated hot grill (broiler) until the cheese begins to brown.

4 Serve with salt and pepper and Dijon mustard.

Reuben's Deli Croque Monsieur

Ingredients

METRIC (IMPERIAL)		AMERICAN
2–3 tablespoons	mayonnaise	2–3 tablespoons
8 slices	rye bread	8 slices
4 thin slices	Gruyere (Swiss) cheese	4 thin slices
4 slices	corned beef	4 slices
1–2 teaspoons	chilli sauce	1–2 teaspoons
100g (4oz)	sauerkraut, rinsed and drained	1 cup
50g (2oz)	butter	¼ cup
2 tablespoons	virgin olive oil	2 tablespoons

Method

1 Spread the mayonnaise over 4 slices of the bread.

2 Cover the remaining slices with layers of cheese, corned beef, chilli sauce and sauerkraut (in that order). Close the sandwiches.

3 Heat the butter and oil in a frying pan (skillet) then cook the sandwiches on both sides until hot and golden brown.

 84   EAT TO BEAT LOW BLOOD SUGAR

Smoked Trout and Feta Cheese Sandwich

Ingredients

METRIC (IMPERIAL)		AMERICAN
4 slices	wholemeal (whole-wheat) bread	4 slices
25g (1oz)	butter or soya margarine	2 tablespoons
2 slices	smoked trout	2 slices
handful	watercress, coarsely chopped	handful
25g (1oz)	feta cheese, crumbled	⅓ cup
4	basil leaves, shredded	4
	salt and freshly ground black pepper	

Method

1 Spread the bread with the butter or margarine.
2 Fill with the smoked trout and top with the watercress.
3 Sprinkle with the feta cheese and basil and season to taste.

Variation

If you prefer, you can make this sandwich with 2 large rolls.

CHAPTER 11

Salads

Bean and Tuna Salad

Ingredients

METRIC (IMPERIAL)		AMERICAN
400g (14oz)	canned flageolet beans, rinsed and drained	2¼ cups
200g (7oz)	canned tuna in olive oil, drained and flaked	1 cup
1	onion, sliced	1
2 tablespoons	chopped fresh parsley	2 tablespoons
	mixed salad leaves, torn into bite-size pieces	

Dressing

	juice of ½ lemon	
3 tablespoons	virgin olive oil	3 tablespoons
	salt and freshly ground black pepper	

Method

1 Place the beans in a mixing bowl. Mix the dressing ingredients together, pour over the beans and mix well.
2 Add the remaining ingredients, except the salad leaves, and gently mix with the beans.
3 Arrange the salad leaves in a serving dish and add the tuna and bean mixture.

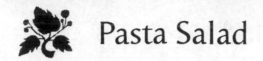

Pasta Salad

Ingredients

METRIC (IMPERIAL)		AMERICAN
225g (8oz)	wholegrain pasta shapes (e.g. fusilli or similar)	½lb
4 tablespoons	fromage frais	4 tablespoons
3 tablespoons	mayonnaise	3 tablespoons
1 tablespoon	white wine vinegar	1 tablespoon
¼ teaspoon	mustard powder	¼ teaspoon
	salt and freshly ground black pepper	
12	radishes, quartered	12
2	celery sticks, finely chopped	2
100g (4oz)	button mushrooms, quartered	1½ cups
1 tablespoon	fresh chives, chopped	1 tablespoon

Method

1 Cook the pasta as directed on the packet, drain and rinse under cold running water.

2 In a mixing bowl blend the fromage frais, mayonnaise, vinegar, mustard and salt and pepper to taste.

3 Stir in the pasta and the remaining ingredients, except the chives. Sprinkle with the chives and serve.

Salade Lyonnaise

Ingredients

METRIC (IMPERIAL)		AMERICAN
225g (8oz)	mixed green salad leaves	½lb
2 slices	granary or wholegrain bread	2 slices
2	garlic cloves, halved	2
8 rashers	streaky bacon, rinded	8 slices
4	eggs	4

Optional

drained canned anchovies, sardines or
  herrings
cooked chicken liver, chopped

Method

1 Tear the salad leaves into bite-size pieces and arrange in 4 individual salad bowls.

2 Toast the bread, gently rub with garlic on both sides, then cut into 2.5cm (1in) cubes.

3 Grill (broil) the bacon until crisp then cut into 2.5 × 5cm (1 × 2in) strips.

4 Add the croutons and bacon to the salad, with any of the optional ingredients if using. Add a dressing to taste and toss.

5 Lightly poach the eggs until they have firm whites but runny yolks, place one on each salad and serve immediately.

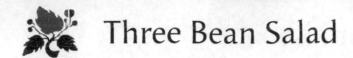

Three Bean Salad

Ingredients

METRIC (IMPERIAL)		AMERICAN
425g (15oz) can	red kidney beans, drained and rinsed	2⅓ cups
425g (15oz) can	borlotti beans, drained and rinsed	2⅓ cups
400g (14oz) can	flageolet beans, drained and rinsed	2¼ cups
1	red onion, sliced	1
1	garlic clove, crushed (minced)	1
1 tablespoon	coriander seeds	1 tablespoon
4 tablespoons	chopped fresh coriander (cilantro)	4 tablespoons
3 tablespoons	virgin olive oil	3 tablespoons
	juice of 1 lime	
	salt and freshly ground black pepper	
225g (8oz)	mixed salad greens or curly-leafed lettuce	½lb

Method

1 Combine the beans, onion and garlic in a large mixing bowl.
2 Dry-fry the coriander seeds then crush with a pestle and mortar. Mix the crushed seeds with the fresh coriander (cilantro) and add to the bowl.
3 Mix the oil and lime juice, season and add to the salad. Mix well and leave to stand for at least 30 minutes, stirring occasionally.
4 Arrange the lettuce in a serving dish, pile the bean salad into the centre and serve.

Warm Bulgar Wheat Salad with Mediterranean-Style Vegetables

This dish serves four as a side dish. If you wish to serve it for two as a main course, add some protein – some spicy sausage would be tasty.

Ingredients

SERVES 4

METRIC (IMPERIAL)		AMERICAN
100g (4oz)	bulgar wheat	⅔ cup
300ml (½ pint)	hot vegetable stock (bouillon)	1⅓ cup
2 small	red (bell) pepper, cored, seeded and quartered	2 small
2 small	aubergine (eggplant), sliced lengthways	2 small
2 small	courgette (zucchini), sliced lengthways	2 small
8 large	chestnut mushrooms, halved	8 large
4 teaspoons	olive oil	4 teaspoons
4	canned artichoke hearts, halved	4
4	sun-dried tomatoes in oil, drained and chopped	4
a few	pitted black olives	a few
2 tablespoons	balsamic vinegar or Vinaigrette Dressing (see page 100)	2 tablespoons
	fresh basil leaves	

Method

1 Soak the bulgar wheat in the stock (bouillon) for 30 minutes. Preheat the oven to 170°C/325°F/gas mark 3. Drain the wheat and place in an ovenproof serving dish. Cover with foil and keep warm in the oven while cooking the vegetables.

2 Lightly brush the pepper, aubergine (eggplant), courgette (zucchini) and mushrooms with olive oil. Grill (broil) for about 10 minutes, turning once, until golden brown on both sides. After 8 minutes, place the artichoke hearts under the grill (broiler) and warm through. Remove all the vegetables from the heat and peel the peppers.

3 Remove the bulgar wheat from the oven and arrange the vegetables on top with any cooking juices from the grill (broiler) pan.

4 Scatter the tomatoes, olives and vinegar or dressing over the vegetables.

5 Garnish with basil and serve at once.

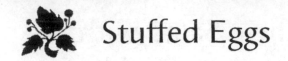

Stuffed Eggs

Ingredients

METRIC (IMPERIAL)		AMERICAN
4 large	eggs, hard-boiled	4 large
2 tablespoons	double (heavy) cream	2 tablespoons
50g (2oz)	blue cheese	½ cup
pinch	salt	pinch
pinch	chilli pepper	pinch
8	anchovy fillets	8
	lettuce leaves	

Method

1 Cut the eggs in half lengthways. Remove the yolks and mash with the cream, cheese, salt and chilli pepper.

2 Pile the filling back into the egg whites and top each half with an anchovy fillet.

3 Serve on a bed of lettuce leaves.

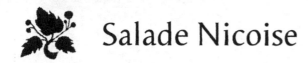

Salade Nicoise

This can be served as a light lunch or main meal.

Ingredients

METRIC (IMPERIAL)		AMERICAN
1	garlic clove, halved	1
225g (8oz)	mixed green salad leaves	½lb
450g (1lb)	tomatoes, quartered	1lb
225g (8oz)	small new potatoes, cooked and quartered	½lb
4	eggs, hard-boiled and quartered	4
100g (4oz)	French beans, lightly cooked	1 cup
12–20	black olives	12–20
5cm (2in)	piece of cucumber, sliced	2in
8	anchovy fillets	8
225g (8oz)	canned tuna in olive oil, drained and flaked	1⅓ cups
	Vinaigrette Dressing (see page 100)	
	fresh parsley or basil, chopped	

Method

1   Rub a salad bowl with the cut garlic, then line the bowl with the salad leaves.
2   In a mixing bowl, combine the tomatoes, potatoes, eggs, beans, olives, cucumber and anchovy fillets.
3   Place the mixture on the salad leaves and sprinkle over the tuna.
4   Dress the salad with the Vinaigrette Dressing and chopped herbs.

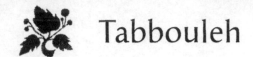

Tabbouleh

Ingredients

METRIC (IMPERIAL)		AMERICAN
225g (8oz)	bulgar wheat	1⅓ cups
1 small	onion, sliced	1 small
1	garlic clove, crushed (minced)	1
50g (2oz)	fresh parsley, chopped	1 cup
	salt and freshly ground pepper	
25g (1oz)	fresh mint, chopped	1 cup
4 tablespoons	lemon juice	4 tablespoons
4 tablespoons	virgin olive oil	4 tablespoons
100g (4oz)	feta cheese or tofu, diced	1⅓ cups
225g (8oz)	tomatoes, sliced	½lb
1 small	cucumber, sliced	1 small
50g (2oz)	black olives, pitted	½ cup

Method

1 Place the wheat in a mixing bowl, cover with cold water and leave to soak for 45–60 minutes.

2 Drain well, return to the mixing bowl and add the onion, garlic and parsley, mixing well. Season to taste.

3 Mix the mint, lemon juice and oil, and pour over the wheat mixture. Stir well and add more lemon juice or seasoning to taste.

4 Place in a large serving dish and sprinkle with the cheese or tofu. Decorate the edge of the salad with the tomatoes, cucumber and olives.

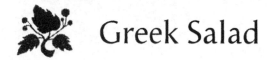

Greek Salad

Ingredients

METRIC (IMPERIAL)		AMERICAN
700g (1½lb)	slicing (beefsteak) tomatoes	1½lb
1	cucumber	1
1 small	lettuce	1 small
2	red onions, thinly sliced	2
125g (4oz)	black olives, pitted	1 cup
225g (8oz)	feta cheese or tofu, diced	2⅔ cups

Dressing

3 tablespoons	lemon juice	3 tablespoons
9 tablespoons	virgin olive oil	9 tablespoons
3 tablespoons	fresh coriander (cilantro), chopped	3 tablespoons
½ teaspoon	fructose	½ teaspoon
	salt and freshly ground black pepper	

Method

1 Chop the tomatoes and cucumber into bite-size chunks.
2 Tear the lettuce leaves into small pieces and place in a large salad bowl.
3 Mix the dressing ingredients well.
4 Add the tomatoes, cucumber, onions and olives to the bowl, and toss well. Pour on the dressing and toss again.
5 Sprinkle with the cheese or tofu and serve.

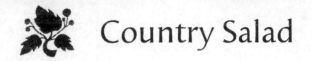

Country Salad

Ingredients

METRIC (IMPERIAL)		AMERICAN
225g (8oz)	asparagus	½lb
25g (1oz)	butter (optional)	2 tablespoons
350g (12oz)	new potatoes, boiled and cooled	¾lb
2	eggs, hard-boiled and cooled	2
1	avocado	1
50g (2oz)	black olives, pitted	½ cup
1 large	courgette (zucchini), sliced	1 large
1 small	red onion, sliced	1 small
3 tablespoons	capers	3 tablespoons
	salt and freshly ground black pepper	
	Vinaigrette Dressing (see page 100)	

Method

1. Steam the asparagus or lightly sauté in the butter until tender. Cut into bite-size chunks.
2. Cut the potatoes and eggs into large slices. Peel and stone the avocado and cut into chunks.
3. Mix the ingredients together in a large serving bowl and add dressing to taste.

Smoked Mackerel Pate Salad

Ingredients

METRIC (IMPERIAL)		AMERICAN
225g (8oz)	smoked mackerel fillets	1⅓ cups
140ml (5fl oz)	natural (plain) bio yogurt	⅔ cup
2 tablespoons	tomato puree (paste)	2 tablespoons
dash of	Worcestershire sauce	dash of
1 tablespoon	fresh parsley, chopped	1 tablespoon
	black pepper	
50g (2oz)	mixed green salad leaves	1 cup

Method

1 In a large bowl, flake the mackerel using a fork.

2 Add the yogurt, tomato puree (paste), Worcestershire sauce, chopped parsley and black pepper to taste. Combine well.

3 Arrange the salad leaves on plates and spoon over the pate.

Vinaigrette Dressing

Ingredients

METRIC (IMPERIAL)		AMERICAN
3 tablespoons	virgin olive oil	3 tablespoons
1 tablespoon	lemon juice or white wine vinegar	1 tablespoon
	salt and freshly ground black pepper	
pinch	mustard powder	pinch
½ teaspoon	fructose	½ teaspoon

Method

1 Put all the ingredients in a screw-top jar and shake vigorously.
2 Use immediately or keep chilled.

Crudites and Dips

Shredded and sliced raw vegetables with dips make a great mid-morning or afternoon snack, which can easily be taken to the office. The vegetables used should be a varied selection of the following:

- baby carrots
- radishes
- strips of fennel
- celery
- spring onions (scallions)
- sliced bell peppers
- cucumber
- cauliflower
- young fresh green beans etc.

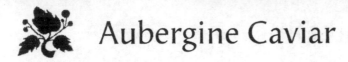

Aubergine Caviar

Ingredients

METRIC (IMPERIAL)		AMERICAN
2	large aubergines (eggplants)	2
	juice of a large lemon	
3 tablespoons	extra-virgin olive oil	3 tablespoons
1 large	garlic clove	1 large
2 tablespoons	natural (plain) bio yogurt	2 tablespoons
	salt and freshly ground black pepper	
5–6	coriander seeds	5–6

Method

1 Heat the oven to 200°C/400°F/gas mark 6. Bake the aubergines (eggplants) whole until they are soft.

2 Cut in half, scoop out the flesh into a bowl and add the lemon juice.

3 Beat in the olive oil, drop by drop, until it forms a smooth cream.

4 Crush the garlic and stir it into the mixture.

5 Stir in the yogurt and season to taste with the salt and pepper.

6 Crush the coriander seeds and add. Stir well once more, then cover the bowl and chill for at least an hour.

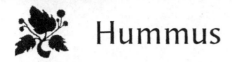

Hummus

Ingredients

METRIC (IMPERIAL)		AMERICAN
425g (15oz)	canned chickpeas, rinsed and drained	2 cups
3 tablespoons	tahini	3 tablespoons
1	garlic clove, crushed (minced)	1
1 tablespoon	sesame oil	1 tablespoon
	juice of ½ lemon	
	a little water to mix (if required)	

Method

1 Put the chickpeas in an electric blender or food processor with the tahini, garlic, sesame oil and lemon juice. Blend until smooth.

2 Add a little water if necessary, so that the mixture is easily spoonable.

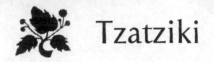

Tzatziki

Ingredients

METRIC (IMPERIAL)		AMERICAN
½	fresh cucumber	½
4	fresh garlic cloves, crushed (minced)	4
	a little sea salt	
300g (10½oz)	strained Greek-style yogurt	1⅓ cups
2 teaspoons	white wine vinegar	2 teaspoons

Method

1 Peel the cucumber and then grate it on a medium-coarse grater. Wrap it in a clean tea towel to remove as much moisture from the cucumber as you can.

2 Place the cucumber in a bowl, add the garlic and salt and combine thoroughly.

3 Add the yogurt and vinegar and combine well again. Serve nicely chilled.

CHAPTER 12

Soups

Parsnip and Sesame Soup

Ingredients

METRIC (IMPERIAL)		AMERICAN
25g (1oz)	soya margarine	2 tablespoons
1 tablespoon	oil	1 tablespoon
1 large	onion, coarsely chopped	1 large
450g (1lb)	parsnips, coarsely chopped	1lb
1 teaspoon	dried rosemary	1 teaspoon
600ml (1 pint)	water	2½ cups
1	bay leaf	1
50g (2oz)	cashew nuts, ground	½ cup
50g (2oz)	sesame seeds, ground	½ cup
600ml (1 pint)	soya milk	2½ cups
300ml (½ pint)	apple juice	1⅓ cups
	salt and freshly ground pepper	
1–2 teaspoons	sesame seeds, toasted	1–2 teaspoons

Method

1 Heat the margarine and oil in a large saucepan and fry the onion for 3–4 minutes until soft but not browned.
2 Stir in the parsnips and rosemary, cover and cook for 4–5 minutes.
3 Add the water and bay leaf, bring to the boil, cover and simmer for 25–30 minutes.
4 Remove the bay leaf and stir in the ground cashew nuts, ground sesame seeds, soya milk and apple juice.
5 Liquidize in a blender or food processor until smooth and creamy (add more apple juice or water if a thinner consistency is desired).
6 To serve, reheat, stirring occasionally. Do not allow to boil. Season to taste and serve garnished with the whole sesame seeds.

Red Lentil, Tomato and Basil Soup

Ingredients

METRIC (IMPERIAL)		AMERICAN
2 tablespoons	sunflower oil	2 tablespoons
1 large	onion, sliced	1 large
1 large	garlic clove, crushed (minced)	1 large
1	bay leaf	1
400g (14oz)	canned chopped tomatoes	2 cups
pinch	dried basil	pinch
1	celery stick, finely chopped	1
175g (6oz)	split red lentils	1 cup
1.4 litres (2½ pints)	vegetable stock (bouillon)	6 cups
	salt and freshly ground black pepper	
	fresh basil	

Method

1 Heat the oil in a large saucepan and fry the onion and garlic until soft but not browned.

2 Add the bay leaf, tomatoes and dried basil and cook for 2 minutes.

3 Stir in the celery, lentils and stock (bouillon). Bring to the boil and continue cooking over a high heat for 15 minutes.

4 Lower the heat and simmer for 20–30 minutes until the lentils are tender.

5 Season to taste and serve garnished with the fresh basil.

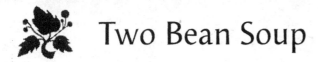

Two Bean Soup

Ingredients

Metric (Imperial)		American
350g (12oz)	dried haricot (navy) beans soaked overnight, drained	¾lb
1.7 litres (3 pints)	water	7½ cups
25g (1oz)	soya margarine	2 tablespoons
2 tablespoons	olive oil	2 tablespoons
3	garlic cloves, crushed (minced)	3
225g (8oz)	onions, chopped	1⅓ cups
225g (8oz)	French beans, chopped	2 cups
1.1 litres (2 pints)	Celery Stock (see page 113)	5 cups
	salt and freshly ground black pepper	

Method

1 Put the beans and water in a large saucepan, bring to the boil, then cover and simmer for about 2 hours or until tender.

2 Heat the margarine and oil in a pan, add the garlic, onion and French beans. Cook gently for a few minutes then gradually add the stock (bouillon). Cover and simmer for 20 minutes.

3 Put half the haricot beans and liquid into a blender, liquidize until smooth and pour into a saucepan.

4 Mix in the remaining beans and liquid, and add the vegetables and their stock (bouillon).

5 Reheat, stirring gently, season and serve.

Chilled Avocado Soup

Ingredients

Metric (Imperial)		American
2 large	ripe avocados	2 large
	juice and grated zest of a lemon	
1	garlic clove, crushed (minced)	1
	salt and freshly ground pepper	
1.4 litres (2½ pints)	unsweetened soya milk	6 cups

Method

1 Peel the avocados, remove the stones and cut the flesh into chunks.

2 Put the chunks in a blender with the lemon juice and zest, garlic and seasoning.

3 Liquidize, then gradually add the milk to make a smooth, thin puree.

4 Chill for at least 1 hour before serving.

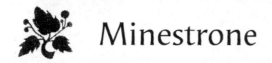

Minestrone

This soup is great favourite of my family and is inspired by the recipe for Minestrone in Claire Macdonald's book Suppers. *It takes time to prepare the vegetables, but it is well worth the effort.*

Ingredients

METRIC (IMPERIAL)		AMERICAN
3 tablespoons	olive oil	3 tablespoons
2	onions, finely chopped	2
6 rashers	back bacon, finely diced or	6 strips
1 packet	cubetti di Pancetta (cubes of Spanish Serrano ham)	1 packet
3	potatoes, peeled and diced	3
225g (½lb)	Brussels sprouts, trimmed and sliced into 3–4 pieces	2 cups
2	carrots, diced	2
3	celery sticks, trimmed and finely sliced	3
420g (15oz) can	chopped tomatoes	2 cups
1.1 litres (2 pints)	chicken or beef stock (bouillon)	5 cups
140ml (¼ pint)	red wine	⅔ cup
1 teaspoon	pesto sauce	1 teaspoon
420g (15oz) can	sugar-free baked beans	2 cups
75g (3oz)	tiny soup pasta (preferably wholegrain)	½ cup
	salt and freshly ground black pepper	
	Parmesan cheese to serve	

Method

1 Heat the olive oil in a large saucepan, add the chopped onions and diced bacon or Pancetta and cook, stirring occasionally, for about 5 minutes. Add the diced potatoes, Brussels sprouts, carrots and celery and continue to cook, stirring from time to time, for several more minutes.

2 Pour in the chopped tomatoes, stock (bouillon), wine and pesto. Let this mixture simmer very gently, with the pan half-covered with its lid.

3 Cook for 25–30 minutes. Before serving stir in the baked beans and pasta, season with salt and pepper and simmer for a further 10 minutes.

4 Serve sprinkled with Parmesan cheese.

Note

Those who wish to avoid meat can use chopped tofu instead of bacon and vegetable stock (bouillon) instead of a meat-based one. The wine can be replaced with extra vegetable stock, if necessary.

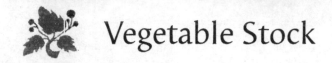

Vegetable Stock

Ingredients

MAKES 1 LITRE (1¾ PINTS) 4½ CUPS

METRIC (IMPERIAL)		AMERICAN
about 225g (8oz)	mixed green vegetable leaves (e.g. cabbage, spinach, Brussels sprouts, cauliflower), chopped	½lb
1 large	onion, chopped	1 large
1 large	carrot, chopped	1 large
1 litre (1¾ pints)	water	4½ cups
	salt and freshly ground black pepper	

Method

1 Place all the ingredients in a large saucepan, bring to the boil, then cover and simmer for 30 minutes.

2 Liquidize all the ingredients in a blender, then cool and strain. The stock keeps for up to 2 weeks in a screw-top bottle in the refrigerator.

Note

The outer leaves of vegetables are the most flavoursome and nutritious, so ensure you include them.

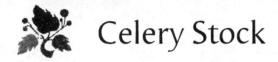

Celery Stock

Ingredients

METRIC (IMPERIAL)		AMERICAN
1	celery head, chopped	1
2	onions, chopped	2
1 litre (1¾ pints)	water	4½ cups
	salt and freshly ground black pepper	
2	garlic cloves, sliced	2
2–3	bay leaves or parsley stalks	2–3

Method

1 Place all the ingredients in a saucepan, bring to the boil and cover and simmer for at least 45 minutes.

2 Crush the vegetables with a potato masher. Allow to cool, then strain. This stock will keep for up to 2 weeks in screw-top bottles in the fridge.

CHAPTER 13

Main meals

Chickpea and Mushroom Curry

Ingredients

METRIC (IMPERIAL)		AMERICAN
3 tablespoons	vegetable oil	3 tablespoons
1 small	onion, chopped	1 small
2	garlic cloves, chopped	2
2 teaspoons	fresh ginger root, chopped	2 teaspoons
1 large	tomato, peeled and chopped	1 large
125ml (4fl oz)	Vegetable Stock (see page 112)	½ cup
400g (14oz)	canned chickpeas, rinsed and drained	2¼ cups
1 tablespoon	mild curry powder	1 tablespoon
1 teaspoon	ground coriander	1 teaspoon
200g (7oz)	rice (optional)	1 cup
225g (8oz)	button mushrooms, quartered	3 cups
40	cashew nuts	40
4 tablespoons	Greek yogurt	4 tablespoons

Optional

2 tablespoons	fresh coriander (cilantro), chopped	2 tablespoons

Method

1 Heat 2 tablespoons of the oil in a pan, add the onion, garlic and ginger, and fry for 5 minutes. Puree in a food processor with the tomato and stock (bouillon) until smooth.

2 Return to the pan and add the chickpeas, curry powder and ground coriander.

3 Bring to the boil, cover and simmer for 20 minutes.

4 If you are including rice, cook it according to the packet instructions.

5 Heat the remaining oil, fry the mushrooms and nuts for 3 minutes then add to the chickpea mixture.

6 Simmer for 5 minutes, stir in the yogurt and coriander (cilantro), heat through and serve with the rice, if desired.

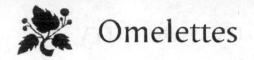

Omelettes

Ingredients

METRIC (IMPERIAL)		AMERICAN
2–3	fresh eggs	2–3
1 tablespoon	water or soya milk	1 tablespoon
	salt and freshly ground white pepper	
knob of	butter or soya margarine	1 tablespoon

Method

1 Break the eggs into a mixing bowl and, using a fork, break the yolks and gently mix the eggs, adding the water or milk and seasoning.

2 Heat an omelette pan or non-stick frying pan (skillet) over a gentle heat. When hot, add the butter or margarine and heat until foaming but not brown.

3 Add the egg mixture. Stir slowly with a wooden spatula, drawing the mixture away from the sides of the pan to the centre as it sets. Let the liquid egg in the centre run to the sides, tilting the pan slightly.

4 When the eggs have set, stop stirring and cook for a further 30 seconds to 1 minute until the omelette is golden brown underneath and still creamy on top. Do not overcook or it will be tough.

5 If making a filled omelette, add the filling at this point. Tilt the pan away from you slightly and use a palette knife to fold over a third of the omelette to the centre of the pan, then fold over the opposite third.

6 Slide the omelette out onto a warm plate. If serving a filled omelette, flip it over so the folded sides are underneath.

7 Serve at once on a warm plate.

OMELETTE FILLINGS

Smoked tofu

Use 25–50g (1–2oz) $\frac{1}{3}$–$\frac{2}{3}$ cup finely sliced smoked tofu.

Spread down the centre of the omelette before folding.

Fine herbs

Use 1 teaspoon mixed dried herbs or 2 teaspoons finely chopped fresh herbs.

Add to the egg mixture before cooking.

Tomatoes

Peel and chop 1–2 tomatoes, place in the centre of the omelette before folding.

Mushrooms

Use 50g (2oz) $\frac{3}{4}$ cup sliced mushrooms. Cook in a separate pan in soya margarine or butter for 5–6 minutes then place in the centre of the omelette before folding.

Cheese

Use 25–50g (1–2oz) $\frac{1}{4}$–$\frac{1}{2}$ cup grated Cheddar cheese. Sprinkle half the cheese down the centre of omelette; the rest of the cheese can be scattered over the finished omelette.

Bacon

Fry 2 rashers (strips) of lean bacon, cut into small pieces and place in the centre of the omelette before folding.

Fish

Gently heat 25–50g (1–2oz) $\frac{1}{4}$–$\frac{1}{3}$ cup of cooked, flaked fish with a little cheese sauce. Place in the centre of the omelette before folding.

Ham

Add 50g (2oz) $\frac{1}{3}$ cup chopped ham and 1 teaspoon of chopped parsley to the omelette mixture before cooking.

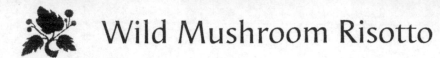

Wild Mushroom Risotto

Ingredients

METRIC (IMPERIAL)		AMERICAN
25g (1oz)	dried porcini mushrooms	⅓ cup
125ml (4fl oz)	boiling water	½ cup
2 tablespoons	olive oil	2 tablespoons
1 small	onion, finely chopped	1 small
350g (12oz)	button mushrooms, halved if large	6 cups
350g (12oz)	arborio rice	1½ cups
1.1 litres (2 pints)	Vegetable Stock (see page 112)	5 cups
15g (½oz)	butter	1 tablespoon
50g (2oz)	Parmesan cheese, grated	½ cup
	salt and freshly ground black pepper	

Method

1 Soak the porcini mushrooms in the boiling water for 15 minutes. Drain and reserve the liquid. Chop the mushrooms.

2 Heat the oil in a large frying pan (skillet), add the onion and cook for 5 minutes until golden.

3 Add the button mushrooms and chopped porcini and cook over a medium heat for 3–5 minutes.

4 Add the rice and cook, stirring for 1 minute, coating all the grains with the mixture.

5 Add 150ml (¼ pint) ⅔ cup of the stock (bouillon) and cook, stirring frequently, until all the stock has been absorbed.

6 Gradually add the remaining stock (bouillon) and reserved porcini liquid until all the liquid has been absorbed.

7 Continue to cook, stirring, for 30 minutes or until the rice is tender with a crunchy middle – 'al dente'. (Do not rush this stage, the rice should have a creamy consistency).

8 Remove the pan from the heat, stir in the butter and cheese, and season to taste. Cover the pan and let it stand for 10 minutes.

9 Stir the mixture again and serve with a crisp salad of mixed leaves.

Vegetarian Lasagne

Ingredients

Metric (Imperial)		American
2	garlic cloves, crushed (minced)	2
2	onions, thinly sliced	2
3 tablespoons	olive oil	3 tablespoons
¼ teaspoon	dried thyme or	¼ teaspoon
1 teaspoon	chopped fresh thyme	1 teaspoon
450g (1lb)	button mushrooms, halved	2½ cups
450g (1lb)	chestnut mushrooms, thickly sliced	2 cups
50g (2oz)	butter or soya margarine	¼ cup
50g (2oz)	wholemeal (whole-wheat) flour	½ cup
600ml (1 pint)	milk	2½ cups
	salt and freshly ground black pepper	
1 teaspoon	freshly grated nutmeg	1 teaspoon
5	sheets no-cook lasagne	5 sheets
225g (8oz)	mozzarella cheese, drained and thinly sliced	½lb
25g (1oz)	Parmesan cheese, grated	¼ cup

Method

1 Preheat the oven to 200°C/400°F/gas mark 6.
2 Fry the garlic and onions in 2 tablespoons of the olive oil for 5 minutes. Add the remaining oil and the thyme and mushrooms, and cook for 30 minutes.
3 Melt the butter in a large pan, add the flour and cook for 1 minute. Gradually add the milk and bring to the boil. Simmer for 1 minute, stirring constantly.
4 Season with salt and pepper and the nutmeg. Set aside 300ml (½ pint) 1⅓ cups of the sauce. Stir the remainder into the mushroom mix.
5 Spread half the mushroom mix onto the base of a 25 × 18 × 5cm (10 × 7 × 2in) ovenproof dish.
6 Cover with half the pasta and repeat the mushroom layer and pasta layer. Pour over the reserved sauce.
7 Cover with the cheese and bake for 30 minutes.

Liver and Bacon Casserole

This is a great family favourite that heralds the beginning of autumn or the log fires of winter.

Ingredients

SERVES 4

METRIC (IMPERIAL)		AMERICAN
2 tablespoons	plain (all-purpose) wholemeal (whole-wheat) flour	2 tablespoons
	salt and freshly ground black pepper	
350g (12oz)	lambs' liver, thinly sliced	1½ cups
2 tablespoons	oil	2 tablespoons
225g (8oz)	onions, thinly sliced	2 cups
4 rashers	streaky bacon, sliced	4 slices
225g (8oz)	carrots, thinly sliced	1½ cups
300ml (½ pint)	beef stock (bouillon)	1⅓ cups

Method

1 Preheat the oven to 180°C/350°F/gas mark 4.
2 Season the flour with the salt and pepper. Coat the liver slices with the seasoned flour.
3 Heat the oil in a frying pan (skillet) and fry the onions for 5 minutes until soft. Add the liver and fry, turning gently, until brown but not totally cooked.
4 Transfer the liver and onions to a casserole and add the bacon and carrots to the frying pan (skillet).
5 Add the stock (bouillon) to the pan and then bring to the boil, stirring constantly. Season to taste.
6 Pour the mixture into the casserole, cover and cook for 1½ hours.

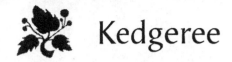

Kedgeree

Ingredients

METRIC (IMPERIAL)		AMERICAN
175g (6oz)	brown rice	¾ cup
450g (1lb)	smoked undyed haddock fillets	1lb
150ml (¼ pint)	skimmed (skim) milk	⅔ cup
2	eggs, hard-boiled and chopped	2
100g (4oz)	frozen petit pois peas	⅔ cup
25g (1oz)	butter	2 tablespoons
	salt and freshly ground black pepper	
	chopped fresh parsley, to garnish	

Method

1 Cook the rice in a saucepan of fast-boiling, salted water for about 25 minutes until tender. Drain well and rinse under cold water.

2 Poach the fish in the milk for 10–15 minutes until tender. Drain, reserving the liquid.

3 Skin and bone the fish, and flake the flesh.

4 Put the flaked fish and rice in a pan, stir in the eggs, peas and little of the fish liquor. Add the butter and season to taste.

5 Cook gently over a low heat until heated through. Serve garnished with parsley.

Stuffed Mushrooms

Ingredients

METRIC (IMPERIAL)		AMERICAN
4 large	field mushrooms, stalks removed and chopped	4 large
50g (2oz)	wholemeal (whole-wheat) breadcrumbs	1 cup
25g (1oz)	walnuts, finely chopped	3 tablespoons
50g (2oz)	Cheddar cheese, grated	½ cup
pinch	dried mixed herbs	pinch
1 tablespoon	sugar-free tomato ketchup	1 tablespoon
	freshly ground black pepper	

Method

1 Preheat the oven to 190°C/375°F/gas mark 5.

2 Place the mushroom caps on a greased baking sheet.

3 Mix the remaining ingredients well, including the mushroom stalks.

4 Spoon the mixture into the mushroom caps.

5 Bake for 10 minutes in the preheated oven.

Soya Bean Burgers

Ingredients

METRIC (IMPERIAL)		AMERICAN
425g (15oz)	canned soya beans, rinsed and drained	2⅓ cups
100g (4oz)	wheatgerm	1 cup
1 small	onion, chopped	1 small
2 medium	eggs, beaten	2 medium
1 tablespoon	soy sauce	1 tablespoon
1	tomato, peeled and pulped	1

Method

1 Preheat the oven to 190°F/375°C/gas mark 5.
2 Mash the beans with a potato masher.
3 Combine all the ingredients in a mixing bowl.
4 Divide the mixture into four, roll into balls and flatten into burger shapes.
5 Place on a greased baking sheet and bake in the preheated oven for 25 minutes.
6 Turn the burgers over, bake for a further 15 minutes and serve.

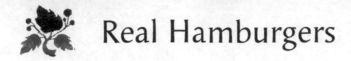

Real Hamburgers

Ingredients

METRIC (IMPERIAL)		AMERICAN
225g (8oz)	minced (ground) beef steak	1 cup
	salt and freshly ground black pepper	
25g (1oz)	butter	2 tablespoons
1 tablespoon	groundnut oil	1 tablespoon
	mixed salad or stir-fried vegetables to serve	

Method

1 Season the beef. Divide into two portions, gently form into balls and flatten into burger shapes.

2 Heat the butter and fry the burgers until crisp on both sides, allowing 3–4 minutes for rare; 5–6 minutes if you like yours more well done. Cut open and check that the meat is done to your liking before serving.

3 Serve with either a tossed mixed salad or stir-fried vegetables.

Variations

Add 2 teaspoons Dijon mustard and 1 teaspoon Worcestershire sauce to the mix.
Alternatively, add 2 tablespoons of chopped fresh parsley and 2 tablespoons grated mature cheese.

Italian Rabbit

I discovered and perfected this recipe whilst spending a couple of months in rural France, where fresh wholesome game was readily available.

Ingredients

SERVES 6

METRIC (IMPERIAL)		AMERICAN
40g (1½oz)	butter	3 tablespoons
6 portions	jointed rabbit	6 portions
130g (4oz)	cubetti di Pancetta or cubes of Spanish Serrano ham	4oz
1	onion, finely chopped	1
6	shallots, finely chopped	6
1	carrot, finely chopped	1
3	garlic cloves, finely chopped	3
300ml (½ pint)	white wine	1⅓ cups
300ml (½ pint)	beef stock (bouillon)	1⅓ cups
1	bouquet garni	1
	salt and freshly ground black pepper	
2 tablespoons	tomato puree (paste)	2 tablespoons
225g (8oz)	mushrooms, quartered	3 cups
2 tablespoons	cornflour (cornstarch)	2 tablespoons
	cooked brown rice or wholegrain pasta, to serve	

Method

1 Melt the butter in a large casserole, add the rabbit, diced ham, onion, shallots, carrot and garlic and saute until the rabbit is browned all over.
2 Add the wine and beef stock (bouillon) to cover, bouquet garni and seasoning.
3 Cover and simmer for 1 hour.
4 Stir in the tomato puree (paste) and mushrooms, and cook for a further 30 minutes.
5 Just before serving, mix the cornflour (cornstarch) with a little water, stir into the casserole and bring to the boil to thicken the mixture.
6 Serve with cooked brown rice or wholegrain pasta.

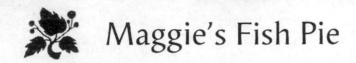

Maggie's Fish Pie

Another popular family dish, this can be jazzed up if guests come for supper by using monkfish, adding smoked (undyed) haddock, salmon or cooked prawns.

Ingredients

METRIC (IMPERIAL)		AMERICAN
700g (1½lb)	cod fillet or mixed white fish fillets and shelled cooked prawns (shrimp)	1½lb
1	bay leaf	1
	salt and freshly ground black pepper	
about 600ml (1 pint)	water	about 2½ cups
50g (2oz)	soya margarine	¼ cup
40g (1½oz)	plain (all-purpose) flour	¼ cup
300ml (½ pint)	soya milk	1⅓ cups
2 tablespoons	fresh parsley, chopped	2 tablespoons
2	eggs, hard-boiled and coarsely chopped	2

Topping

450g (1lb)	potatoes, boiled and mashed with a little butter	1lb
40g (1½oz)	Cheddar cheese, grated	⅓ cup

Method

1 Place the cod (or other fish) in a large pan, add the bay leaf, salt, pepper and enough water to cover. Poach gently for about 10–15 minutes.

2 Remove the fish with a slotted spoon, strain and reserve the cooking liquid. Remove and discard the skin and bones from the fish and flake the flesh.

3 In a small pan, melt the margarine, add the flour and stir together. Heat gently for 2 minutes, stirring constantly.

4 Gradually blend in the milk and about 150ml (¼ pint) ⅔ cup of the reserved fish liquor. If using prawns (shrimp), add them at this stage.

5 Bring to the boil and simmer for 2 minutes, stirring until a smooth sauce has formed.

6 Add the flaked fish, parsley and hard-boiled eggs. Season to taste.

7 Pour the mixture into a pie dish, cover with the mashed potato and sprinkle with the cheese.

8 Place under a preheated hot grill (broiler) until golden brown and crisp.

Maggie's Chicken Cacciatora

This dish is popular in my family, especially on Boxing Day as a way of using up any leftover turkey.

Ingredients

SERVES 4

METRIC (IMPERIAL)		AMERICAN
25g (1oz)	butter	2 tablespoons
½ tablespoon	oil	½ tablespoon
2	celery sticks, sliced	2
1	onion, chopped	1
225g (8oz)	tomatoes, peeled and chopped or	½lb
400g (14oz)	canned chopped tomatoes	2 cups
1	garlic clove, crushed	1
	salt and freshly ground black pepper	
pinch	cayenne	pinch
350g (12oz)	cooked chicken (or turkey), diced	¾lb
75g (3oz)	long-grain brown rice	¾ cup
600ml (1 pint)	chicken stock (bouillon)	2½ cups
	Parmesan cheese, grated	

Method

1 Place the oil and butter in a frying pan (skillet), add the celery, onion, tomatoes and garlic and fry until nearly tender. Season with salt, pepper and cayenne.

2 Add the chicken and allow to heat through.

3 Meanwhile, cook the rice in the stock (bouillon) for about 30 minutes or until the rice is tender and most of the liquid is absorbed.

4 Place the rice on a warmed serving dish, top with the chicken mixture and sprinkle with the Parmesan cheese.

CHAPTER 14

Desserts

Raspberry Mousse

Ingredients

Metric (Imperial)		American
3 teaspoons	gelatine	3 teaspoons
250g (9oz)	low-fat vanilla yogurt	1 cup
2 × 200g (7oz) tubs	low-fat French vanilla fromage frais	1½ cups
4 large	egg whites	4 large
150g (5oz)	fresh or frozen and thawed raspberries, mashed	1½ cups
	fresh raspberries and mint leaves to garnish	

Method

1 Sprinkle the gelatine in an even layer over 1 tablespoon of water in a small bowl and leave to go spongy. Bring a small pan of water to the boil, remove from the heat and place the bowl in the pan. Stir until clear and dissolved.

2 In a large bowl, stir the vanilla yogurt and fromage frais together, then add the gelatine and mix well.

3 Using an electric whisk, beat the egg whites until stiff peaks form, then fold through the yogurt mixture. Transfer half to a separate bowl and fold the mashed raspberries through.

4 Divide the raspberry mixture between the bases of 4 tall glasses or serving bowls. Top with the vanilla mixture. Refrigerate for several hours, or until set.

5 Decorate with the fresh raspberries and mint leaves.

Apple and Hazelnut Yogurt

Ingredients

METRIC (IMPERIAL)		AMERICAN
125ml (4fl oz)	natural unsweetened apple juice	½ cup
450g (1lb)	apples, cored and sliced	1lb
450ml (¾ pint)	natural (plain) yogurt	1¾ cups
1 teaspoon	lemon zest, grated	1 teaspoon
50g (2oz)	hazelnuts, toasted and chopped	½ cup

Method

1 Place the apple juice and apple slices in a pan, bring to the boil and simmer gently for 5–10 minutes.

2 Allow to cool, put into a blender, add the yogurt and blend together.

3 Put the mixture into a serving dish and stir in the lemon zest and hazelnuts.

4 Chill well before serving.

Date and Banana Ice Cream

Ingredients

METRIC (IMPERIAL)		AMERICAN
225g (8oz)	dried dates, pitted	½lb
600ml (1 pint)	water	2½ cups
1	vanilla pod (bean)	1
6 tablespoons	vegetable oil	6 tablespoons
100g (4oz)	soya milk powder	1 cup
3	bananas, peeled and sliced	3

Method

1   Place the dates, water and vanilla pod in a pan, bring to the boil, then cover and simmer for 15–20 minutes until the dates are very soft.
2   Allow the mixture to cool a little then remove and discard the vanilla pod (bean).
3   Pour the dates into a blender, add the remaining ingredients and liquidize until smooth and creamy.
4   Either freeze in an ice-cream maker or transfer to a plastic container and freeze for at least 2–3 hours before serving.

Baked Stuffed Peaches

Ingredients

METRIC (IMPERIAL)		AMERICAN
4 large	ripe peaches	4 large
75g (3oz)	ground almonds	¾ cup
3 tablespoons	fresh orange juice	3 tablespoons
150ml (5fl oz)	natural unsweetened orange juice	⅔ cup

Method

1 Preheat the oven to 190°C/375°F/gas mark 5.

2 Slice round the middle of each peach and gently ease the peach halves away from the stone.

3 Mix the almonds and fresh orange juice to a stiff mixture, then stuff the peaches and replace the tops.

4 Stand the peaches in an ovenproof dish and pour in the unsweetened orange juice.

5 Bake in the preheated oven for 30 minutes until tender.

6 Leave to cool for 5–10 minutes. Place in individual serving dishes and spoon over a little of the cooking juices.

Dried Fruit Compote

A useful dessert for the winter months when few fresh fruits are at their best.

Ingredients

METRIC (IMPERIAL)		AMERICAN
50g (2oz)	dried pears	⅓ cup
50g (2oz)	dried prunes	⅓ cup
50g (2oz)	dried apricots	⅓ cup
50g (2oz)	dried peaches	⅓ cup
50g (2oz)	dried apples	⅓ cup
3	cloves	3
1	cinnamon stick	1
	grated zest of 1 large orange	

Method

1. Place the dried fruit in a saucepan, add enough water to cover and bring to the boil.
2. Remove from the heat, then cover and leave to stand for 1 hour.
3. Drain the fruit, reserving 450ml/15fl oz/2 cups of the juice. Return the fruit to the pan, add the juice, cloves and cinnamon stick and bring to the boil.
4. Simmer gently for 30 minutes until the fruit is soft. Leave to cool.
5. Serve chilled, sprinkle with the orange zest.

Banana Bread Pudding

Ingredients

METRIC (IMPERIAL)		AMERICAN
100g (4oz)	fresh wholemeal (whole-wheat) breadcrumbs	2 cups
1 large	banana, thinly sliced	1 large
75g (3oz)	mixed dried fruit	½ cup
25g (1oz)	soya margarine	2 tablespoons
300ml (½ pint)	milk	1⅓ cups
½ teaspoon	almond essence (extract)	½ teaspoon
50g (2oz)	flaked almonds	½ cup

Method

1 Preheat the oven to 200°C/400°F/gas mark 6.
2 Grease a pie dish then cover the bottom with one-third of the breadcrumbs. Top with half the banana slices and half the dried fruit.
3 Repeat the layering, finishing with a final layer of breadcrumbs.
4 Dot the surface with the margarine.
5 Mix the milk with almond essence (extract), pour over the pudding and sprinkle with the flaked almonds.
6 Bake in the preheated oven for 25–30 minutes until golden brown.

Baked Apples Stuffed with Figs

Ingredients

METRIC (IMPERIAL)		AMERICAN
4 large	cooking apples	4 large
50g (2oz)	dried figs, finely chopped	⅓ cup
50g (2oz)	mixed coarsely chopped nuts	½ cup
25g (1oz)	sunflower seeds	¼ cup
25g (1oz)	butter or soya margarine	2 tablespoons
150ml (5fl oz)	natural unsweetened apple juice	⅔ cup

Method

1 Preheat the oven to 190°C/375°F/gas mark 5.

2 Core the apples and score a slit around the middles to prevent bursting.

3 Mix the figs, nuts and sunflower seeds together and stuff into the apples.

4 Place the apples in a shallow ovenproof dish, dot a little butter or margarine over each apple, then pour over the apple juice.

5 Bake in the preheated oven for 30–35 minutes until soft.

CHAPTER 15

Between-meal snacks and drinks

Peanut and Raisin Cookies

Ingredients

Metric (Imperial)		American
50g (2oz)	soya margarine	¼ cup
100g (4oz)	raisins, minced	⅔ cup
50g (2oz)	smooth peanut butter	½ cup
4 tablespoons	water	4 tablespoons
1 teaspoon	pure vanilla extract	1 teaspoon
1	egg	1
200g (7oz)	81 per cent wholemeal (whole-wheat) flour	1¾ cups
½ teaspoon	baking powder	½ teaspoon
1 teaspoon	bicarbonate of soda (baking soda)	1 teaspoon
a little	skimmed (skim) milk	a little
50g (2oz)	salted peanuts, chopped	½ cup

Method

1 Preheat the oven to 170°C/325°F/gas mark 3.

2 Put the margarine, raisins and peanut butter in a mixing bowl and mix well.

3 Add the water, vanilla and egg, beating well.

4 Mix in the flour, baking powder and bicarbonate of soda (baking soda).

5 Place teaspoons of the mixture on a baking tray, flatten each one and brush with some milk.

6 Press the chopped peanuts into each cookie, then bake in the preheated oven for 15 minutes until golden.

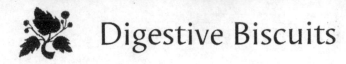
Digestive Biscuits

Ingredients

Metric (Imperial)		American
25g (1oz)	butter, melted, plus extra for greasing	2 tablespoons
100g (4oz)	quick-cook polenta	1 cup
½ teaspoon	salt	½ teaspoon
350ml (12fl oz)	boiling water	1½ cups
1 teaspoon	sesame oil	1 teaspoon
25g (1oz)	sesame seeds	¼ cup

Method

1 Preheat the oven to 200°C/400°F/gas mark 6.
2 Grease 2–3 baking sheets with a little butter.
3 Put the polenta and salt in a heatproof bowl, add the boiling water and stir vigorously until smooth.
4 Stir in the butter and sesame oil. The mixture should have the consistency of thin cream; if it doesn't, add cold water as required.
5 For each biscuit, spoon 1 tablespoon of the mixture onto a baking sheet and spread to make a thin circle – about 4–5 per sheet. Sprinkle with sesame seeds.
6 Bake in batches in the preheated oven for 20–25 minutes until the edges begin to turn brown and crisp.
7 Transfer to a wire rack to cool.

Cheese Crunchies

Ingredients

METRIC (IMPERIAL)		AMERICAN
100g (4oz)	81 per cent wholemeal (whole-wheat) flour	1 cup
40g (1½oz)	soya margarine	3 tablespoons
50g (2oz)	Cheddar cheese, grated	½ cup
½ teaspoon	mustard powder	½ teaspoon
1	egg yolk	1
1½ tablespoons	water	1½ tablespoons

Method

1 Preheat the oven to 180°C/350°F/gas mark 4.
2 Put the flour and margarine in a mixing bowl and mix with a fork.
3 Add the cheese and mustard powder and mix well. Stir in the egg yolk and water.
4 Knead the mixture to form a stiff dough, then chill for 15 minutes.
5 Roll out the dough on a floured surface to 5mm (½in) thickness and cut into 5cm (2in) diameter biscuits.
6 Place on a greased baking tray and bake in the preheated oven for about 15 minutes. Do not allow to overcook.
7 Transfer to a wire rack to cool.

Nutty Oat Biscuits

Ingredients

METRIC (IMPERIAL)		AMERICAN
50g (2oz)	ground almonds	½ cup
75g (3oz)	rolled oats	¾ cup
25g (1oz)	desiccated (shredded) coconut	⅓ cup
25g (1oz)	soya margarine	2 tablespoons
2 tablespoons	pear and apple spread	2 tablespoons
½ teaspoon	pure vanilla extract	½ teaspoon

Method

1 Preheat the oven to 170°C/325°F/gas mark 3.
2 Place all the ingredients in a mixing bowl, mix and combine well.
3 Divide the mixture into 16 equal pieces and roll each one into a ball.
4 Place the balls on a greased or non-stick baking tray and press your thumb into the middle of each ball.
5 Bake in the preheated oven for 10–12 minutes until golden.
6 Transfer to a wire rack to cool.

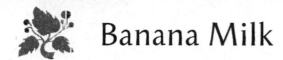

Banana Milk

Ingredients

METRIC (IMPERIAL)		AMERICAN
1 small	ripe banana, sliced	1 small
1	egg	1
1 tablespoon	skimmed (skim) milk powder	1 tablespoon
1 tablespoon	fructose	1 tablespoon
1 teaspoon	smooth peanut butter	1 teaspoon
1 litre (1¾ pints)	soya milk	4½ cups

Method

1 Place the banana, egg, milk powder, fructose and peanut butter in a blender with 300ml (½ pint) 1⅓ cups of the soya milk.

2 Blend until smooth, then add the remaining soya milk.

3 Serve hot or cold.

4 Keep any remaining mixture in a glass screw-top container in the refrigerator.

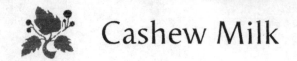

Cashew Milk

Ingredients

METRIC (IMPERIAL)		AMERICAN
100g (4oz)	cashew nuts	1 cup
1 litre (1¾ pints)	water	4½ cups

Method

1 Place the ingredients in a blender and blend for 2 minutes.

2 Keep chilled in a glass screw-top container.

Note

As cashew nuts are naturally sweet you should not need to add flavourings.

Seed and Nut Milk

Ingredients

METRIC (IMPERIAL)		AMERICAN
25g (1oz)	sunflower seeds	¼ cup
75g (3oz)	blanched almonds	¾ cup
650ml (23fl oz)	water	3 cups
1 tablespoon	fructose	1 tablespoon
300ml (½ pint)	soya milk	1⅓ cups
pinch	salt	pinch

Method

1 Place the seeds, nuts and 300ml (½ pint) 1⅓ cups of the water in a blender. Allow to soak for 15–20 minutes, then blend until smooth.

2 Add the fructose, remaining water, soya milk and salt and blend until well mixed.

3 Keep chilled in a glass, screw-top container.

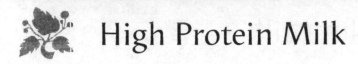

High Protein Milk

Ingredients

METRIC (IMPERIAL)		AMERICAN
2	eggs	2
75ml (2½fl oz)	natural (plain) yogurt	⅓ cup
1 tablespoon	soya oil	1 tablespoon
1 litre (1¾ pints)	water	4½ cups
125g (4oz)	soya flour	1 cup
125g (4oz)	skimmed (skim) milk powder	2⅓ cups

Method

1 Place the eggs, yogurt and oil in a blender and blend until smooth.

2 Add the remaining ingredients and blend until well mixed.

3 Keep chilled in a glass screw-top container.

Egg and Soya Drink

Ingredients

METRIC (IMPERIAL)		AMERICAN
½ tablespoon	soya oil	½ tablespoon
1	egg yolk	1
75ml (2½fl oz)	natural (plain) yogurt	⅓ cup
75ml (2½fl oz)	skimmed (skim) milk	⅓ cup
75ml (2½fl oz)	soya milk or	⅓ cup
12g (½oz)	soya flour	⅛ cup
75ml (2½fl oz)	fresh orange juice (or other fresh fruit juice)	⅓ cup
450ml (¾ pints)	milk	2¼ cups

Method

1 Place all the ingredients in a blender and blend until smooth.

2 Keep chilled in a glass screw-top container.

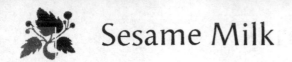

Sesame Milk

Ingredients

METRIC (IMPERIAL)		AMERICAN
100g (4oz)	sesame seeds	¾ cup
1 litre (1¾ pints)	water	4 cups
	fructose to taste (optional)	

Method

1 Place all the ingredients in a blender, blend for 2 minutes then strain well.
2 Keep chilled in a glass screw-top container.

Quick Breakfast Drink

Ingredients

METRIC (IMPERIAL)		AMERICAN
300ml (10fl oz)	natural (plain) yogurt	1⅓ cups
300ml (10fl oz)	fresh orange juice	1⅓ cups
1 large	banana, sliced	1 large
2	egg yolks	2

Method

1 Place all the ingredients in a blender and blend until smooth.
2 Serve very cold with ice.

Quick Protein Drink

Ingredients

METRIC (IMPERIAL)		AMERICAN
300ml (10fl oz)	soya milk	1⅓ cups
2	eggs	2
300ml (10fl oz)	fresh orange juice	1⅓ cups

Method

1 Place all the ingredients in a blender and blend until smooth.

2 Serve chilled.

CHAPTER 16

Baking

Quick and Easy Bread

Ingredients

METRIC (IMPERIAL)		AMERICAN
300g (10oz)	wholemeal (whole-wheat) flour	3 cups
100g (4oz)	soya flour	1 cup
1 teaspoon	fructose	1 teaspoon
2 teaspoons	salt	2 teaspoons
25g (1oz)	soya margarine	2 tablespoons
7g (¼oz)	sachet easy-bake (instant) yeast	½ tablespoon
300ml (½ pint)	tepid water	1⅓ cups

Method

1   Put the flours, fructose and salt in a mixing bowl. Rub (cut) in the margarine then add the dried yeast and mix well.
2   Mix in the water to make a soft dough.
3   Place the dough on a floured surface and knead well for at least 10 minutes, until firm, elastic and non-sticky.
4   Divide the dough in half, shape into rounds, then cover and leave in a warm place for at least 30 minutes or until doubled in size. Meanwhile, preheat the oven to 230°C/450°F/gas mark 8.
5   Place the dough rounds on a greased baking sheet and bake in the preheated oven for 15 minutes. Reduce the heat to 200°C/400°F/gas mark 6 and cook for a further 20–30 minutes.
6   Cool on a wire rack.

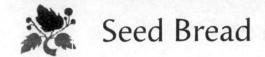

Seed Bread

Ingredients

METRIC (IMPERIAL)		AMERICAN
25g (1oz)	fresh yeast	2 tablespoons
750ml (1¼ pints)	hand-warm water	3¼ cups
1.4kg (3lb)	whole-wheat flour	3lb
50g (2oz)	poppy seeds	⅓ cup
50g (2oz)	sesame seeds	⅓ cup
50g (2oz)	sunflower seeds	⅓ cup
125ml (4fl oz)	soya oil	⅔ cup
¼ teaspoon	salt	¼ teaspoon

Method

1 Put yeast and water in a large bowl and mix until dissolved. Stir in enough flour to make a thick batter. Cover and leave in a warm place for 30 minutes.

2 Stir in the seeds, oil and salt, mix well and slowly add more flour, stirring constantly. When the dough begins to firm, place on a floured surface and knead. Add more flour until the consistency is smooth and elastic.

3 Return the dough to the bowl and leave in a warm place for 1 hour.

4 Gently knead the dough again, divide into three pieces and knead again briefly.

5 Fit the dough into 3 greased and floured 450g (1lb) bread tins (pans), cover and leave to rise for 20–25 minutes. Meanwhile, preheat the oven to 230°C/450°F/gas mark 8.

6 Bake in the preheated oven for 15 minutes. Reduce the heat to 180°C/350°F/gas mark 4 and bake for a further 30 minutes.

7 Remove the bread from the tins (pans) and cool on a wire rack.

High Protein Loaf

Ingredients

METRIC (IMPERIAL)		AMERICAN
6	eggs, separated	6
1 tablespoon	sesame seeds or caraway seeds	1 tablespoon
½ teaspoon	salt	½ teaspoon
225g (8oz)	soya flour, sifted	2 cups

Method

1 Preheat oven to 180°C/350°F/gas mark 4.
2 Beat the egg yolks until very thick and pale. Add the seeds and salt.
3 Beat the egg whites until very stiff, then fold in the yolks. Carefully fold the flour into the mixture.
4 Pour the mixture into a buttered 1kg/2lb loaf tin (pan).
5 Bake for 25 minutes, then reduce the heat to 130°C/250°F/gas mark ½ and bake for a further 15 minutes.
6 Remove from the tin (pan) and cool on a wire rack.

Note

This bread is rather crumbly with a fine sponge-like texture (rather like Madeira cake), and is delicious toasted.

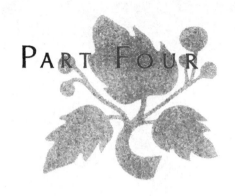

PART FOUR

Taking it Further

CHAPTER 17

Supplement use

The regulation of sugar metabolism involves various glands and organs, chiefly the thyroid, pituitary and adrenal glands, and the liver and pancreas. It therefore follows that anything contributing to a malfunction or deficiency in these organs may also be a causative factor in hypoglycaemia.

There are certain specific substances that play an important role in sugar metabolism. When these nutrients are over- or under-supplied, the organs and glands involved in sugar metabolism may become over- or under-active. These minerals and vitamins are usually prescribed in conjunction with the corrective diet to speed up the normal activity of the sugar-regulating mechanism, and to minimize some of the unpleasant symptoms suffered by the hypoglycaemic patient.

Minerals
Zinc
There is a close relationship between zinc and insulin. It has been shown that zinc can delay the absorption of glucose, leading, in some cases, to reactive hypoglycaemia. Zinc is also involved in the regulation of insulin release.

Chromium
Although chromium is a trace element and present in very small amounts in our diet, it is nonetheless of considerable importance in hypoglycaemia. In 1955, it was identified as the so-called 'glucose tolerance factor', and a deficiency of this mineral has been shown to produce altered glucose tolerance. In 1968, it was observed that glucose tolerance tests showed improvement in elderly patients by the simple addition of chromium to their diet. An interesting bonus achieved by taking chromium is its effect on cholesterol control. Research has shown that chromium can produce a drop of around 14 per cent in the blood cholesterol when added in relatively small amounts to the diet.

Calcium

Calcium has a role in the proper utilization of many minerals, as well as vitamins D, A and C. The most abundant mineral in the body, it plays a part in nerve and muscle control, bone health, blood clotting and heart function. It works closely with magnesium and phosphorous, the correct ratio of the three plus the availability of copper, zinc, manganese and boron is essential to our health.

Magnesium

Magnesium is the main cell constituent mineral after potassium. It plays an important role in sodium, potassium and calcium distribution. It is involved in many enzyme systems and cell functions, and is usually included in supplements for low blood sugar. Its deficiency can lead to liver damage. It is used to treat liver problems, heart disease, pre-menstrual syndrome, joint and muscle problems, high blood pressure, ME, diabetes and epilepsy.

Potassium

Large doses of potassium are of value in treating a diabetic patient who has 'hypo-ed' or when a hypoglycaemic patient experiences a low blood sugar episode (with symptoms of anxiety, palpitations, dizziness, cold sweating and so on); 1g of soluble potassium chloride (available without prescription at most pharmacies and known as Sando-K) taken at this time often quickly relieves the symptoms. The stress produced by hypoglycaemia causes large amounts of potassium to be lost in the urine, mainly owing to adrenal exhaustion. The potassium chloride quickly makes up this deficiency, raises the blood sugar level and reduces the hypoglycaemic symptoms.

I find that a daily dose of 200mg of soluble potassium chloride is adequate with the 1g reserved for acute symptom reactions. (This emergency treatment is of particular benefit when dealing with nocturnal anxiety and is safer and more effective than the usual medical prescription of glucose tablets or sedatives).

Manganese

This mineral plays a vital role in glucose tolerance, being essential for carbohydrate and protein metabolism. The level of manganese is often low in blood and hair mineral analysis results, largely due to current intensive farming and food processing practices that lead to soil depletion. A high manganese intake reduces iron absorption, and a high level of dietary iron inhibits manganese absorption. This highlights the need for caution when taking any mineral supplements, unless a deficiency has been shown in blood tests.

Vitamins

Pantothenic acid (Vitamin B5)

Adrenal exhaustion and hypoglycaemia are very closely linked, the common factor being the frequent lack of pantothenic acid in both conditions. Research has shown that even a slight deficiency of pantothenic acid leads to a decrease in adrenal efficiency with a subsequent imbalance in the sugar metabolism. Deficiency in this B vitamin also affects the insulin-glucose balance, causing the blood sugar to fall very rapidly when insulin is given. As I have said previously, the speed of fall is of the utmost importance in hypoglycaemia.

The vitamin B family

It is normal to prescribe a good high potency vitamin B complex for those with hypoglycaemia. They are of value in many areas of metabolism, aiding vitality, assisting assimilation of fats and, to some extent, reducing the harmful effects of stress on the different organs and tissues. The B vitamins also serve to normalize sugar metabolism. Vitamins B6 and B12 are of special value in helping the adrenal glands, pancreas and the liver to normalize. Biotin assists fatty acid and glucose metabolism, while B3 (Niacinamide) reduces adrenal exhaustion and stress-induced hypoglycaemia.

Vitamin E

This vitamin plays a unique role in circulation and tissue repair. It is of specific value in encouraging the uptake of glucose (as glycogen) in the muscles, thus improving the symptoms of hypoglycaemia.

Vitamin C

The vitamin C requirement is often high when the adrenal glands are overworked or exhausted. This vitamin is also of value in normalizing insulin production.

G.T.F. Complex™

After treating low blood sugar patients for several years, I became aware of the need to have access to a specific multi-formula to prescribe for low blood sugar. The UK company Nutri (who only deal directly with practitioners) agreed to produce the G.T.F. Complex™ to my formula. Many vitamins and minerals are vital to the function of the G.T.F. and the information overleaf provides readers with some idea of the nutrients and dosages involved.

Each capsule typically contains:

Magnesium (citrate)	33.33mg	Thiamin HCL	8.34mg
Vitamin C (as ascorbic acid)	166.67mg	Manganese (aspartate)	1.67mg
Potassium (aspartate)	33.34mg	Riboflavin	8.33mg
Calcium (citrate)	16.67mg	PABA	8.33mg
Vitamin E (as d-alpha acetate)	66.67mg	Zinc (aspartate)	2.5mg
Pantothenic Acid (as pantothenate)	41.67mg	Vanadium (vanadyl sulphate)	380ug
Vitamin B12 (as cyanocobalamin)	42ug	Pituitary (anterior) (Bovine)	1.67mg
Choline (bitartrate)	16.67mg	Chromium (nicotinate)	33.34ug
Adrenal (freeze dried) (Bovine)	33.34mg	Parotid (freeze dried) (Bovine)	1.67mg
N-Acetyl-Cysteine	16.67mg	Folacin (as folic acid)	50ug
Niacin (as niacinamide)	16.67mg	Biotin	0.016mg
Inositol	16.67mg		
Vitamin B6 (as pyridoxine HCL)	8.34mg		

Encapsulated with gelatin, Ascorbyl Palmitate

The usual prescription is 2–6 capsules daily, depending upon the severity and age of the patient being treated. The G.T.F. Complex™ is not recommended during pregnancy or breast-feeding. It is also not recommended for children under 12 years of age unless directed by a health care professional.

The G.T.F. Complex™ contains an adrenal glandular extract. As some confusion and controversy surrounds the value of glandular products, I shall briefly outline their history and use.

RAW GLANDULAR THERAPY

Animal tissue concentrates, also termed protomorphogens or organ-specifics, have been in use for thousands of years. The basis of the therapy is that like cures like i.e. that animal glands can provide the appropriate nutrient proportions that are found in our own organs and glands. The glands are taken from non-European free-range cattle. After removal, the glands are de-fatted and kept frozen until processed. The glandular preparations in current use are referred to as 'raw' because no heat is used in their processing.

The critics of raw glandulars (or 'cow parts' as they have named them) argue that they fail to be clinically effective because material contained in the glands is reduced to basic amino acids (the building blocks of protein) in the process of digestion, and therefore do not possess any specific therapeutic value. The glandular detractors argue that those who take glandular supplements would obtain the same 'benefits' by eating any type of protein, for instance, fish, meat, cheese or eggs.

In addition, they claim that unless proteins are broken down into simple amino acids they cannot be absorbed from the gut and passed into the bloodstream, as they would be too large. There is evidence that when enzymes and proteins are absorbed through the gut lining, approximately 50 per cent passes into the blood. Significantly this is in the form of molecules that have not been reduced to amino acids. Leon Chaitow, in his book *The Raw Materials of Health*, states that 'Furthermore, and of critical significance to the concept of using specific organs and glands in therapy, it is known that at least 20 per cent of these unchanged (by digestion) protein molecules retain their original characteristics'. It seems likely therefore that when raw glandular supplements are properly prepared from stress-free, healthy, free-range animals they provide a specific therapeutic value for the gland that is targeted.

The nutritional make-up of the glands and organs of animals are chemically very similar to their human counterparts. It follows, therefore, that the specific nutritional constituents that are provided by such a system will be in the optimum ratios and quantities.

Bovine Spongiform Encephalopathy (BSE)

Concern has been expressed over the risk of BSE when taking glandular products. Reassurance has been offered by Nutri on its glandular products with the following statement: 'All glandular material of bovine source used in Nutri products is sourced from grass-fed, Argentinian range cattle or from US/Canadian pasture-fed or corn-fed cattle. The cattle are never fed meat-derived meal as per United States Department of Agriculture (USDA) rules and regulations. The USDA and the US Food and Drug Administration (FDA) approve all procedures concerned with the use of glandular material. The USDA state that BSE has no history in the USA, Canada or Argentina.'

I have prescribed glandular products to support adrenal, thyroid and pancreatic metabolism for many years and have never identified any side-effects or adverse effects on patients' health.

Specific supplements for vegetarians and vegans

Many patients who avoid animal products in their diet are understandably resistant to the use of the G.T.F. Complex™ and other glandular supplements. Fortunately, a vegetarian alternative is available – UltraGlycemX™ (also produced by Nutri). This powdered drink can be used for treating all types of dysglycaemia – and it's suitable for vegetarian and vegan diets. It provides support for those with poor glucose metabolism, when combined with a low blood sugar diet. It offers high-quality protein, carbohydrates and fat, with specific vitamins, minerals and other nutrients to nutritionally support insulin/glucose tolerance.

UltraGlycemX™ is free of dairy, lactose, wheat, gluten, egg, yeast, artificial colours and artificial flavours. It can be used as a balanced supplement or it can be taken as a meal replacement for those who are overweight. Its constituents include Vitamins A, B, C, D and E, and the minerals, calcium, phosphorous, magnesium, copper, zinc, chromium, manganese and selenium. It also contains high levels of the antioxidant alpha lipoic acid.

Essential fatty acids (EFAs)

Also known as omega-3 and omega-6, these are of value in maintaining normal blood sugar. The EFAs play a role in glucose tolerance and insulin control and sensitivity. Insulin resistance can be reduced by including EFAs in our diet, thus reducing the likelihood of obesity, high blood pressure, dysglycaemia, elevated blood fats, fatigue and low blood sugar. Although food is always the preferred source of the essential fatty acids, they are widely available in capsule form from health stores and pharmacies.

Omega-3

This family of fatty acids is deficient in the Western diet. The chief sources include cold-water fish and fish oil supplements (salmon, trout, sardines, mackerel and eel). Fish oil can be destroyed by high temperatures and significantly the Japanese (who have enviably low levels of heart disease) often eat fish raw in the form of sushi or sushimi. Flax seed oil and to a lesser extent walnut and rapeseed, or canola, oil also contain the omega-3 EFAs.

Omega-6

These EFAs are found chiefly in safflower, sunflower and corn oil, sesame and sunflower seeds, and evening primrose oil, borage oil and blackcurrant seed oil. Excessive consumption of the omega-6 EFAs can serve to depress the omega-3 EFAs.

All the essential fatty acids are important, but a balance of the two is important for a healthy diet. In his best-selling book *Dr Atkins Vita-Nutrient Solution*, Dr Atkins writes 'What is becoming inescapably clear is that the essential fatty acids are collectively the number one missing nutrient in the American diet'.

Glossary

Adrenal glands

Two glands, located adjacent to the top of each kidney. The glands consist of two portions, the cortex and the medulla. The cortex secretes cortisol (hydrocortisone), cortisone and adrenal androgens. The androgens serve as precursors to testosterone and oestrogens. The medulla secretes adrenaline (epinephrine) and noradrenaline (norepinephrine).

Adrenaline

Also known as epinephrine. A hormone produced by the adrenal glands to facilitate sudden physical activity in an emergency, and to raise the blood sugar level.

Adrenocortex stress profile

A test that measures the adrenal hormones cortisol (hydrocortisone) and DHEA (Dehydroepiandrosterone) in the saliva. The test consists of four saliva samples taken over a 24-hour period.

Body Mass Index (BMI)

Recommended weight/height ratio. Calculated by dividing your weight in kilograms by the square of your height in metres. A healthy BMI is usually between 20 and 25.

Calorie

The amount of heat required to raise the temperature of one gram of water by 1°C. The total amount of heat available from full combustion of food is 4.1 Kcal per gram from carbohydrates, 4.3 Kcal per gram from protein, and 9.0 Kcal per gram from fat.

   Note: in nutritional and metabolic studies the Kilocalorie is generally abbreviated to Calorie but written with a capitol C to indicate that it is the larger unit.

Carbohydrate

Energy-producing compounds of carbon, oxygen and hydrogen (starch, sugar, glucose etc.)

Carnitine

An amino acid used to reduce blood fat levels and heart disorders – often referred to as the 'fat-burner'. Found mainly in red meat, it requires the co-factors iron and vitamin C to prevent a deficiency.

Cholesterol

A fat-soluble substance occurring in animal fats, oils and egg yolks. It is found in the bile, blood, brain tissue, liver, kidneys, adrenal glands and nerves, and is a precursor of steroid and sex hormones including cortisol, cortisone, DHEA, progesterone, oestrogen and testosterone. Cholesterol can crystallize in the gall bladder to form gallstones. Only 20 per cent of the total cholesterol is dietary, the remaining 80 per cent being produced by the liver.

Cortisol (hydrocortisone)

A steroid hormone produced by the adrenal cortex. Its functions include glucose metabolism and protein and fat regulation. It assists in regulation of the immune system.

Cortisone

A steroid hormone involved in carbohydrate and protein regulation. It can be converted into cortisol. However, most of the cortisone found in the body is formed from cortisol.

DHEA (dehydroepiandrosterone)

A 'mother' hormone, made from cholesterol and released by the adrenal glands. The precursor hormone of many steroid and sex hormones.

Dysglycaemia

Any derangement of the sugar content of the blood.

Dysinsulinism

Term implying disturbance of normal insulin-production. It can result in a combination of high and low blood sugar, usually considered to be pre-diabetic.

Endocrine

Means literally secreted internally, and is applied to substances produced and released into the blood, especially hormones.

Endocrine system

A network of glands that secrete hormones directly into the bloodstream. These include the pituitary, the thyroid, the adrenals and the pineal gland.

Enzyme

An enzyme is a protein substance that catalyses chemical reactions of various substances without itself being destroyed or altered. Although many enzyme reactions occur within cells, digestive enzymes operate outside the cells in the digestive tract.

Epinephrine

see Adrenaline

Essential Fatty Acids (EFAs)

Polyunsaturated acids including linoleic, alpha-linolenic and archidonic. EFAs are, as their name suggests, essential for growth, maintenance and function of body cells. They are also necessary for the normal functioning of the reproductive and endocrine systems and for the breaking up of cholesterol deposits on arterial walls. Sources include safflower, soya, olive and corn oils, fish oils and poultry fat and game. (*see* Omega).

Fructose

Fruit sugar, also called levulose. Found in all sweet fruits.

Functional, or reactive, hypoglycaemia

see Hyperinsulinism

Gastritis

Inflammation of the stomach lining.

Glandular extracts

see Protomorphogens

Glucose Tolerance Factor (GTF)

A nutritional compound consisting of chromium, vitamin B3 and the amino acids (proteins) glycine, glutamic acid and cysteine. Because of its importance in the Glucose Tolerance Factor, chromium is itself often referred to as GTF Chromium.

Glucose Tolerance Test (GTT)

A two-, five- or six-hour test involving frequent blood glucose measurements after the ingestion of 50–100gm (2–4oz) of soluble glucose. The GTT is used as an aid to the diagnosis of diabetes and hypoglycaemia.

Glycaemic Index (GI)

A method devised to assess foods according to the extent that they increase the blood sugar. The higher the GI of a food, the speedier it increases the blood sugar. Many factors influence a food's GI number, including sugar content and type, and fibre content. The GI has many inconsistencies, and different lists show differing numbers for the same foods. Generally speaking, the lower the number the better the food for health and weight control. However, a food's GI listing only indicates a given food's effect on our blood sugar – it does not take food quality or nutritional value into account.

HDL cholesterol (High density lipoproteins)

The 'good' cholesterol. This plasma protein is made in the liver and contains about 50 per cent protein with cholesterol and triglycerides. It is involved in transporting cholesterol and other fats from the body. The cholesterol passes from cells to the liver, where it is converted to bile, which passes into the intestines and is eliminated in our stools.

Histamine

A substance found in the body that is released after injury, allergy or inflammation; also involved in the control of tissue permeability.

Hydrocortisone

see Cortisol

Hyperinsulinaemia

see Hyperinsulinism

Hyperinsulinism

Inappropriately high levels of insulin in the blood. Also defined as insulin resistance. Elevated blood insulin leads to calories being converted to fat instead of energy. Hypoglycaemia can also result from insulin excess.

Hyperthyroidism

Hyperactivity of the thyroid gland. This can accelerate all the metabolic processes of the body.

Hypoglycaemia

Inappropriately low level of blood glucose. Usually caused by adrenal hypofunction or an insulin excess (as in diabetes control or hyperinsulinism).

Hypothyroidism

Underactivity of the thyroid gland.

Insulin

Hormone released by the islet glands of the pancreas to control the level of sugar in the blood.

Insulin resistance

A term used to define the effects of a typical high-sugar, refined-carbohydrate Western diet. The high level of sugar it contains leads to insulin overproduction and fat storage. Many who suffer from late onset diabetes do not have an insulin deficiency but a tendency to be insensitive to the effects of insulin. Their cells do not respond effectively to the insulin message and their blood sugar rises. The blood insulin levels also rise as the body attempts to balance the blood sugar.

Ketogenic diet

High fat/protein diet, with low carbohydrates prescribed to encourage weight loss through breakdown of body's fat reserves.

Lactose

Milk sugar – breaks down to galactose and glucose.

Leaky gut syndrome

Increased gut permeability. This can allow the leakage of toxic substances from the gut into the bloodstream. Chronic gut inflammation caused by Candida albicans and other parasites can cause a leaky gut.

Low blood sugar

see Hypoglycaemia

LDL (Low Density Lipoprotein) cholesterol

The 'bad' cholesterol that carries cholesterol and fats (triglycerides) from foods and our liver to our cells.

Omega-3 and omega-6

The essential fatty acids. Omega-3 is found in fish oils (from cold water fish), flax seed oil, soya bean oil, walnut oil and wild game. The chief sources of omega-6 are safflower oil, sunflower oil and corn oil. Evening primrose oil, starflower oil and blackcurrant seed oil are also sources of omega-6.

Pancreas

Gland situated in the left upper abdomen, which secretes digestive enzymes and insulin (when used for food, the pancreas of an animal is known as a sweetbread).

Paratoid glands
Pair of salivary glands located at the side of the face, just below and in front of the external ear.

Pituitary gland
A vital endocrine gland in the skull, responsible for control of the other endocrine glands such as the adrenals, thyroid and ovaries.

Pregnenolone
Sometimes called the 'grandmother' hormone because other hormones, including DHEA, oestrogen, testosterone, cortisol and progesterone, are synthesized from pregnenolone. An adrenal steroid hormone, it is prescribed for depression and rheumatic symptoms.

Protomorphogens (glandular extracts)
Animal (usually bovine) glands used for treating a variety of illnesses. The centuries-old practice of using specific tissue has been found beneficial for adrenal, thymus, thyroid, ovarian, pituitary and other gland and organ deficiencies. These 'organ-specific' nutrients provide safe, specific nutritional support to failing or imbalanced glands and organs.

Raw glandular therapy
see Protomorphogens

Reactive hypoglycaemia
see Hypoglycaemia

Syndrome X (metabolic syndrome)
A disorder characterized by a number of conditions, including obesity, high blood pressure, raised blood fats and insulin resistance. Considered a risk factor in heart disease and adult onset diabetes.

Transient hypoglycaemia
Temporary low blood sugar, usually due to exercise, fatigue or missed meals. Usually reversible without treatment.

Triglycerides
Stored body fat, derived from the diet or synthesized in the liver.

Resources

Buying organic fruit and vegetable boxes
The Soil Association
Bristol House
40–56 Victoria Street
Bristol
BS1 6BY
Tel: 0117 929 0661
Web: www.soilassociation.org
Email: info@soilassociation.org

Buying local produce
National Association of Farmers' Markets
South Vaults
Green Park Station
Green Park Road
Bath
BA1 1JB
Tel: 01225 787 914
Web: www.farmersmarkets.net
email: nafm@farmersmarkets.net

Countryside Alliance Food Co-operatives
Sharron Rourke
Rural Regeneration Manager
Unit 5c
Lakeland Business Park
Cockermouth
Cumbria
CA13 0QT
Tel: 01900 828 870
Email: sharron-rourke@countryside-alliance.org

Supermarket contacts
ASDA
Tel: 0500 100 055
Web: www.asda.co.uk
Email: customer.services@asda.co.uk

Co-op
Tel: 0800 317 827
Web: www.co-op.co.uk
Email: customer.relations@co-op.co.uk

Iceland
Tel: 01244 842 675
Web: www.iceland.co.uk
Email: customer.care@iceland.co.uk

Marks & Spencer
Tel: 020 7268 1234
Web: www.marksandspencer.com
Email: customer.care@marks-and-spencer.com

Wm Morrison
Tel: 01924 870 000
Web: www.morrisons.plc.uk

Sainsbury's
Tel: 0800 636 262
Web: www.sainsburys.co.uk
Email: bsh@tao.sainsburys.co.uk

Safeway
Tel: 01622 712 987
Web: www.safeway.co.uk
Email: feedback@safeway.co.uk

Somerfield/Gateway/Kwiksave
Tel: 0117 935 6669
Web: www.somerfield.co.uk
Email: gill.baker@somerfield.co.uk

Tesco
Tel: 0800 505 555
Web: www.tesco.co.uk/indexn.htm
Email: customerservice@tesco.co.uk

Waitrose
Tel: 0800 188 884
Web: www.waitrose.co.uk
Email: customer_service@waitrose.co.uk

THE AUTHORS MAY BE CONTACTED AT:

Ridge Cottage
29 Ferncroft Road
Bournemouth
Dorset
BH10 6BY
Web: www.martin-budd.com
e-mail: mlb@martin-budd.com
(Please enclose a stamped self-addressed envelope)

Index

CPSIA information can be obtained
at www.ICGtesting.com
Printed in the USA
LVHW060759280719
625415LV00007B/14/P